Navigating Life with Parkinson's Disease

Lisa M. Shulman, MD

Editor-in-Chief, *Brain & Life®* Books Series
Fellow of the American Academy of Neurology
Professor of Neurology
The Eugenia Brin Professor in Parkinson's Disease and Movement Disorders
The Rosalyn Newman Distinguished Scholar in Parkinson's Disease
Director, University of Maryland Parkinson's Disease and
Movement Disorders Center
University of Maryland School of Medicine
Baltimore, MD

Other Titles in the *Brain & Life®* Books Series

Navigating Life with a Brain Tumor
Lynne P. Taylor, MD, FAAN; Alyx B. Porter Umphrey, MD; and Diane Richard

Navigating the Complexities of Stroke
Louis R. Caplan, MD, FAAN

Navigating Life with Multiple Sclerosis
Kathleen Costello, MS, ANP- BC, MSCN; Ben W. Thrower, MD;
and Barbara S. Giesser, MD

Navigating Life with Epilepsy
David C. Spencer, MD, FAAN

Navigating Life with Amyotrophic Lateral Sclerosis
Mark B. Bromberg, MD, PhD, FAAN, and Diane Banks Bromberg, JD

Navigating Life with Migraine and Other Headaches
William B. Young, MD, FAAN, FANA, FAHS and Stephen D. Silberstein, MD,
FAHS, FAAN, FACP

Navigating Life with Chronic Pain
Robert A Lavin, MD, MS, Sara Clayton, PhD, and Lindsay Zilliox, MD

Navigating Life with Parkinson's Disease

Second Edition

Sotirios A. Parashos, MD, PhD

Struthers Parkinson's Center
HealthPartners Park Nicollet
Golden Valley and St. Paul, MN;
Allied Team Training Program Parkinson's Foundation and
Department of Neurology
University of Minnesota
Minneapolis, MN

Rose L. Wichmann, PT

Struthers Parkinson's Center
HealthPartners Park Nicollet
Golden Valley and St. Paul, MN

AMERICAN ACADEMY OF
NEUROLOGY.

OXFORD
UNIVERSITY PRESS

OXFORD

UNIVERSITY PRESS

Oxford University Press is a department of the University of Oxford. It furthers
the University's objective of excellence in research, scholarship, and education
by publishing worldwide. Oxford is a registered trade mark of Oxford University
Press in the UK and certain other countries.

Published in the United States of America by Oxford University Press
198 Madison Avenue, New York, NY 10016, United States of America.

© American Academy of Neurology 2020

First Edition published in 2012
Second Edition published in 2020

Library of Congress Cataloging-in-Publication Data
Names: Parashos, Sotirios A., author. | Wichmann, Rose L., author
Title: Navigating life with Parkinson's disease / Sotirios A. Parashos and Wichmann, Rose L.
Description: Second edition. | New York : Oxford University Press, 2020.
Series: Brain and life books |
Includes bibliographical references and index.
Identifiers: LCCN 2019048533 (print) | LCCN 2019048534 (ebook) |
ISBN 9780190877477 (paperback) | ISBN 9780190877491 (epub)
Subjects: LCSH: Parkinson's disease—Patients. |
Parkinson's disease—Patients—Rehabilitation. | Self-care, Health.
Classification: LCC RC382 .P3497 2020 (print) | LCC RC382 (ebook) |
DDC 616.8/33—dc23
LC record available at https://lccn.loc.gov/2019048533
LC ebook record available at https://lccn.loc.gov/2019048534

This material is not intended to be, and should not be considered, a substitute for medical or
other professional advice. Treatment for the conditions described in this material is highly
dependent on the individual circumstances. And, while this material is designed to offer
accurate information with respect to the subject matter covered and to be current as of the
time it was written, research and knowledge about medical and health issues are constantly
evolving and dose schedules for medications are being revised continually, with new side
effects recognized and accounted for regularly. Readers must therefore always check the
product information and clinical procedures with the most up-to-date published product
information and data sheets provided by the manufacturers and the most recent codes of
conduct and safety regulation. The publisher and the author make no representations or
warranties to readers, express or implied, as to the accuracy or completeness of this material.
Without limiting the foregoing, the publisher and the author make no representations or
warranties as to the accuracy or efficacy of the drug dosages mentioned in the material. The
author and the publisher do not accept, and expressly disclaim, any responsibility for any
liability, loss, or risk that may be claimed or incurred as a consequence of the use and/or
application of any of the contents of this material.

Printed in Canada by Marquis Book Printing

CONTENTS

Here is a question for you:

If you know more about your neurologic condition, will you do better than if you know less?

Well, it's not only optimism but also hard data that show that individuals who are more knowledgeable about their medical conditions *do have better outcomes,* so learning about your neurologic condition plays an important role in doing the very best you can. The main purpose of both the American Academy of Neurology's (AAN's) *Brain & Life* Patient Books and *Brain & Life* magazine is to focus on the needs of people with neurologic disorders. Our goal is to view neurologic issues through the eyes of people with neurologic problems in order to understand and respond to their practical day-to-day needs.

So, you are probably saying, "Of course, knowledge is a good thing, but how can it change the course of my disease?" Well, health care is really a two-way street. You need to find a knowledgeable and trusted neurologist; however, no physician can overcome the obstacle of working with inaccurate or incomplete information. Your physician is working to navigate the clues you provide in your own words combined with the clues from their neurologic examination to arrive at an accurate diagnosis and respond to your individual needs. Many types of important clues exist, such as your description of your symptoms or your ability to identify how your neurologic condition affects your daily activities. Poor patient–physician communication inevitably results in less-than-ideal outcomes. This problem is well described by the adage, "garbage in, garbage out." The better you pin down and communicate your main problem(s), the more likely you are to walk out of your doctor's office with the plan that is right for you. Your neurologist is the expert in your disorder, but you and your family are the experts in you. Physician decision-making is not a "one-size-fits-all" enterprise, yet when accurate, individualized information is lacking, that's what it becomes.

Whether you are startled by hearing a new diagnosis or you come to this knowledge gradually, learning that you have a neurologic problem is jarring. Many neurologic disorders are chronic; you aren't simply adjusting to something new—you will need to deal with this disorder for the foreseeable future. In certain ways, life has changed. Now, there are two crucial "next steps": The first is finding good neurologic care for your problem, and the second is successfully adjusting to living with your condition. This second step depends on attaining knowledge of your condition, learning new skills to manage the condition, and finding the flexibility and resourcefulness to restore your quality of life. When successful, you regain your equilibrium and restore a sense of confidence and control that is the cornerstone of well-being.

When healthy adjustment does not occur following a new diagnosis, a sense of feeling out of control and overwhelmed often persists, and no doctor's prescription will adequately respond to this problem. Individuals who acquire good self-management skills are often able to recognize and understand new symptoms and take appropriate action. Conversely, those who are lacking in confidence may respond to the same symptom with a growing sense of anxiety and urgency. In the first case, watchful waiting or a call to the physician may result in resolution of the problem. In the second case, the uncertainty and anxiety often lead to multiple physician consultations, unnecessary new prescriptions, social withdrawal, or unwarranted hospitalization.

Outcomes can be dramatically different depending on knowledge and preparedness.

Managing a neurologic disorder is new territory, and you should not be surprised that you need to be equipped with new information and a new skill set to effectively manage your condition. You will need to learn new words that describe both your symptoms and their treatment to communicate effectively with the members of your medical team. You will also need to learn how to gather accurate information about your condition when you need it and to avoid misinformation. Although all your physicians document your progress in their medical records, keeping a personal journal about your neurologic condition will help you summarize and track all your medical information in one place. When you bring this journal with you as you go to see your physicians, you will be able to provide more accurate information about your history and previous treatment. Your active and informed involvement in your care and decision-making results in better quality of care and better outcomes.

Your neurologic condition is likely to pose new challenges in daily activities, including interactions in your family, workplace, and social and recreational activities. How can you best manage your symptoms or your medication dosing schedule in the context of your normal activities? When should you disclose your diagnosis to others? *Brain & Life* Patient Books provide you with the background you need, including the experiences of others who have faced similar problems, to guide you through this unfamiliar terrain. Our goal is to give you the resources you need to "take your doctor with you" when you confront these new challenges. We are committed to answering the questions and concerns of individuals living with neurologic disorders and their families in each volume of the *Brain & Life* Patient Books. We want you to be as prepared and confident as possible to participate with your doctors in your medical care. Much care is taken to develop each book with you in mind. A special authorship model takes a multidisciplinary team approach to put together the most up-to-date, informative, and useful answers to the questions that most concern you—whether you find yourself in the unexpected role of patient or caregiver. Each authorship team includes neurologists with special expertise along with a diversity of other contributors with special knowledge of the particular neurologic disorder. Depending on the specific condition, this includes rehabilitation specialists, nurses, social workers, and people or family members with important shared experiences. Professional writers work to ensure that we avoid "doctor talk," and easy-to-understand definitions of new terms appear on the page when a new word is introduced. Real-life experiences of patients and families are found throughout the text to illustrate important points. And, feedback based on correspondence from *Brain & Life* magazine readers informs topics for new books and is integral to our quality improvement. These new features will be found in all books in the *Brain & Life* Patient Books so that you can expect the same quality and patient-centered approach in every volume.

I hope that you have arrived at a new understanding of why knowledge is empowering when it comes to your medical care and that *Brain & Life* Patient Books will serve as an important foundation for the new skills you need to be effective in managing a neurologic condition.

Lisa M. Shulman, MD, FAAN
Editor-in-Chief, *Brain & Life*® Patient Books
and Professor of Neurology
University of Maryland School of Medicine

FOREWORD FROM THE FIRST EDITION

As mortals with finite life spans, we unconsciously recognize that middle age and beyond will be associated with medical conditions. However, when confronted with an age-related neurologic "disease" we tend to panic. This is especially true with Parkinson's disease, which has gained much publicity in recent years. Famous athletes have become disabled with this condition, and relatives or friends may be in nursing homes with Parkinson's disease.

Knowledge about their condition is crucial to people with any major disorder, and certainly this is true for Parkinson's disease. The early panic and initial despair at the diagnosis can be tempered by knowledge. Parkinson's disease compromises lives, but it is treatable. With optimal treatment, people with Parkinson's disease can often lead quite normal lives for many, many years. Obviously, this varies among individuals, but the diagnosis should not be regarded as a death sentence. For example, in Olmsted County, Minnesota (where I live), people with Parkinson's disease live to ages within 3 years of the life spans that would be predicted without the disease.

The primary author of this book, Dr. Sotirios Parashos, and the other contributors are to be congratulated for writing this comprehensive text for people with Parkinson's disease and their families.

It was written under the auspices of the American Academy of Neurology, a physician organization that demands fair and balanced works. They have addressed all the fundamental issues that confront individuals with Parkinson's disease, defining terms and providing a balanced discussion. In the present era of electronic media and the Internet, we are constantly confronted with medical "facts." Moreover, it is easy to use a search engine to find information about virtually anything, including Parkinson's disease. Of course, the problem with the lay press is that the medical information is not always vetted. The Internet dogmatically provides all sorts of information, but how much of it is true? Consequently, an unbiased and comprehensive book for people with Parkinson's disease is crucial, and this text provides a myriad of information that will serve the Parkinson's disease community well.

As you read this book, be reassured by the fact that Parkinson's disease is treatable; the goal for clinicians such as me is to keep people in the mainstreams of their lives. As you will read, exercise and activity are very important for people with Parkinson's disease, and optimum medical treatment is therefore crucial to allow such exercise. Philosophies about Parkinson's disease treatment vary among clinicians. This is evident if you use the US National Library of Medicine search engine, PubMed; enter the search term "Parkinson's disease treatment," and approximately 34,000 published articles surface. If you scan some of the more recent entries, you will realize that treatment approaches are quite varied. The authors of this book needed to be cognizant of those differing approaches while avoiding legitimization of marginal therapies. Thus the treatment chapters take a very comprehensive view of what is available and how clinicians of disparate therapeutic philosophies might select specific drugs or therapies. This background will be invaluable for patients when interacting with their personal clinicians and also when reading Internet entries.

Family and caregivers are important members of the Parkinson's disease team. Knowledge about this condition will help them understand the lifestyle compromises that surface to variable extents over the course of this disorder. As we age, we all will need family and caregivers, and for those with Parkinson's disease this is especially true. They also will appreciate this book.

J. Eric Ahlskog, MD, PhD

Consultant in Neurology, Mayo Clinic;

Professor of Neurology,

Mayo Clinic Alix School of Medicine, Rochester, MN;

Author of another Oxford University Press book for those with Parkinson's disease: *The Parkinson's Disease Treatment Book: Partnering with Your Doctor to Get the Most from Your Medications*

PREFACE FROM THE FIRST EDITION

In an era where information on just about everything that has to do with health and illness is for many people only a few keystrokes away, it is only natural to ask, "Why one more book about Parkinson's disease?"

The reasons for this undertaking are multiple but have a lot to do precisely with the fact that information about Parkinson disease is abundant and accessible. For people recently diagnosed with the disease and their loved ones, it quickly becomes a daunting task just to navigate through all this information, not to mention to be able to sort out the reliable from the not-so-reliable sources. For people in the more advanced stages of the disease who seek specific answers to their specific problems, there can very easily be too much information. It is great news that research has expanded our understanding of Parkinson disease in the last decade, but it has also created a maze of possibilities and directions that is very hard to follow, quite often even for the scientists and physicians who have dedicated their lives in the fight to conquer this disease.

Considering the "lay of the land," it would be irrational to even suggest that the book in your hands constitutes a comprehensive review of the disease. It can, however, be a good compass both to the uninitiated and to the "old hands." The text will take you through the basics of Parkinson's, the theories about its causes, the symptoms of its various stages, and the available treatments, including medications, therapies, and brain surgery. More importantly, whole chapters are dedicated to day-to-day management of the disease symptoms, strategies to improve function and ameliorate quality of life, and even legal and financial advice. A number of resources are cited so that the interested reader can seek further information through reliable, authoritative websites. The information presented in this book is accompanied by illustrative examples and true stories relating experiences of persons with Parkinson's and their care partners. We have asked Parkinson's experts to give us their "2 cents" on some "hot topics," and these vignettes are easily identifiable and set apart from the main text for easy access and reference. For more practical items, we adopted a question-and-answer format for easy assimilation of the information.

This book was truly a group effort. We would like to thank our expert panel for their knowledgeable insights and the persons with Parkinson's and their care partners who were very kind to share their experiences for this book. We would like to thank Dr. Brent Clark of the University of Minnesota for providing us with photographs of the Lewy body and the substantia nigra. We also thank Rick Vandendolder, OTR, of the Struthers Parkinson's Center for his help with photographing adaptive equipment for people with Parkinson's. Dr. Lisa Shulman, series editor, and Ms. Andrea Weiss of the *Neurology Now* series were very supportive throughout this effort. Craig Panner of Oxford University Press can be credited for making sure the book made sense as a whole and has been particularly helpful, patient, and accommodating throughout the process of publishing the book.

Last but not least, we would like to thank the Parkinson disease community, a very proactive group of people, who make our efforts so much easier with their support and dedication to our common goal.

PREFACE TO THE SECOND EDITION

It is hard to believe it has been only 8 years since the publication of our first edition. In this short time, so much has changed in what we know about Parkinson's disease and how to treat it. As I read through the first edition, I found much information was already out of date within 4 years from publication. More than 200 years after the publication of Parkinson's *An Essay on the Shaking Palsy* and just over 50 years after the implementation of levodopa in Parkinson's treatment, it looks as though scientists are poised to make a breakthrough toward effective treatments of the disease itself, not just the symptoms, and paths that may eventually lead to a cure are now visible. Such progress would be impossible without the hard work of many researchers; the financial support of the corresponding government agencies; the advocacy of national and international Parkinson's organizations and the philanthropy of their donors; and the tireless efforts and open minds of the doctors, nurses, therapists, and social workers caring for people with Parkinson's and their families. Above all, none of this progress would be possible without the active participation of people with Parkinson's and their families through advocacy, community engagement, and participation in clinical trials. To them we would like to extend a great "thank you."

In the second edition, we have added what is new in our understanding of the mechanisms that underlie the pathology in Parkinson's disease and how this new knowledge has shaped our understanding of disease progression, symptom evolution, and quest for a cure; new developments in the diagnostic process; new information on the use of genetics in understanding and possibly treating the disease more effectively; new medications and improved use of older medications to treat both the motor and nonmotor symptoms of the disease; new information on complementary therapies and the use of medical cannabis; new information on the use of technology to manage symptoms better; and new websites and Internet resources. We also asked more people with Parkinson's to share their stories and experiences. Our thanks go out once again to everyone who helped with the first edition and were happy to help with this second effort, including Craig Panner and his team at Oxford University Press and, more than ever, the people with Parkinson's and their families who contributed their stories and experiences and continue to teach us and inspire our efforts.

Navigating Life with Parkinson's Disease

CHAPTER 1

Introduction

In this chapter, you will learn about

- The main symptoms of Parkinson's
- Some famous people who lived with Parkinson's
- How to use this book

Terry plays basketball on weekends. For a few weeks, he had noticed an occasional slight tremor in his right hand, which he thought was strange because he didn't remember banging it during a game. Then he noticed that sometimes the tiny shaking in his hand occurred when he walked. And sometimes it happened when he wasn't doing anything—he'd just be standing, his arm at his side, and the trembling, ever so mild, would begin. Terry, a healthy man in his mid-40s, didn't give any of this much thought. He was too busy with his life; during the day, he had a challenging job as an executive at a successful advertising agency, and at home, he enjoyed relaxing with his wife. One morning, he got out of bed to go to the bathroom and his wife saw his right hand shaking. It wasn't pronounced, but it was a definite shake. She talked to Terry about it, and he told her about other times it had happened. They decided he should go see a doctor. After an examination, Terry's doctor told him he had **Parkinson's disease** (Parkinson's for short).

Like Terry, about 1.5 million Americans are living with Parkinson's disease. Older people are more likely to get Parkinson's disease than younger people: the average age of diagnosis is 67. But about 15 percent of people with Parkinson's begin showing symptoms before the age of 50, and the disease can be seen in much younger people. About two out of every hundred people older than 70 are living with Parkinson's disease. The disease affects both men and women and people of all ethnic groups.

Parkinson's disease is named for James Parkinson, a London physician who wrote the book *An Essay on the Shaking Palsy* (Figure 1.1) about the illness in 1817. Originally called "shaking palsy" or "paralysis

AN

ESSAY

ON THE

SHAKING PALSY.

BY

JAMES PARKINSON,
MEMBER OF THE ROYAL COLLEGE OF SURGEONS.

LONDON:
PRINTED BY WHITTINGHAM AND ROWLAND,
Goswell Street,
FOR SHERWOOD, NEELY, AND JONES,
PATERNOSTER ROW.
1817.

FIGURE 1.1 Frontispiece of James Parkinson's "An Essay on the Shaking Palsy."

agitans," it was later renamed Parkinson's disease by Charcot, a famous French **neurologist** of the nineteenth century. In his book, Parkinson defined the condition he had observed in patients this way: "Involuntary tremulous motion, with lessened muscular power, in parts not in action and even when supported; with a propensity to bend the trunk forward, and to pass from a walking to a running pace: the senses and intellects being uninjured." Through the years, we have come to recognize that the main target of Parkinson's disease is in the brain. Normally, a small cluster of nerve cells (or **neurons**) called the **substantia nigra**, which is located in the brainstem, produces **dopamine**, a chemical that is essential to smooth movement. Parkinson's is a neurodegenerative disorder. The word **neurodegenerative** indicates a premature death of neurons. In Parkinson's disease, the dopamine-producing (or **dopaminergic**) neurons of the substantia nigra die prematurely. For this reason, the brains of people with Parkinson's are deficient in dopamine, and the result is loss of smooth, full-range motion. However, as the disease progresses, more and more brain structures become involved in the degenerative process. In the later stages of the disease, other brain functions besides movement are affected, causing many of the so-called nonmotor symptoms of the disease. What's more, there are new theories about where the process starts, years before it reaches the substantia nigra. Knowledge gained in the past years may well shine new light on both causes and a path to better treatments, even a possible cure. More on this later.

The exact cause of Parkinson's disease is unknown: despite years of research, we still don't understand what kills these dopaminergic neurons. Some researchers have identified certain environmental factors that may increase one's chances of developing the disease. An example of such environmental influences is exposure to pesticides and other chemicals that are common on farms and ranches: North Dakota (one of the most rural areas in the United States) has the highest rate of Parkinson's disease in the nation. In some people, the cause of Parkinson's disease can be found in their **genes**.

Early motor signs of Parkinson's disease include smaller handwriting, a soft voice, reduced facial expression, slowness of movement, tremor, and changes in walking (shuffling) and posture (stooping). Not all people with Parkinson's have all these symptoms. To be diagnosed with Parkinson's disease, a person needs to exhibit at least two of the four cardinal symptoms: **tremor, bradykinesia** (slowed movement), **rigidity**, and **postural instability**. Because the diagnosis is difficult to make, some specialists have proposed that Parkinson's disease cannot be diagnosed unless bradykinesia is one of the two symptoms. Some people who will develop Parkinson's disease later in life may lose their sense of smell early on, sometimes even decades before they ever experience any tremor, rigidity, or bradykinesia. Others may suffer from a peculiar sleep disorder in which they act out their dreams while they are still asleep. Many people with Parkinson's have a lifelong history of constipation. These early symptoms that may lead to Parkinson's disease later in life may offer new clues about where and how the disease starts.

Currently, a movement disorders specialist will consider a number of "diagnostic criteria" when making the diagnosis of Parkinson's disease. These were developed several years ago by the International Parkinson and Movement Disorder Society, an international society of clinicians who treat people with Parkinson's. Some of these criteria may be important features or findings on physical examination, while others may be diagnostic tests, such as specialized brain scans. Some criteria are necessary to make the diagnosis, others are "supportive" but not necessary, and yet another group is "exclusionary" criteria, which means that if these features are present, they point away from the diagnosis of Parkinson's disease.

Parkinson's disease happens because of the premature death of dopamine-producing nerve cells in the **substantia nigra**. The exact cause of the disease is unknown.

Parkinson's is a remarkably individualized disease. Nearly every person's story is different. One person may experience tremor at the early stages of the disease, while another may experience tremor at a later stage of the disease or even not at all; in others, new symptoms may replace tremor as the disease progresses. One of the things that is true for all people with Parkinson's is that the disease progresses over time. In the beginning, a person may have only a few symptoms, but new symptoms will usually develop later. The dopamine-producing neurons will continue to die, the amount of dopamine in the brain will continue to decline, and a person's symptoms will become worse. Depending on a wide variety of factors—including age, severity of the illness, medication, and exercise—some people may experience more intrusive, sometimes even disabling, symptoms over years or decades. Others may have a very slow progression of the symptoms and can live very productive lives without any significant impairment.

The Cardinal Symptoms of Parkinson's Disease Explained

- **Tremor:** Shaking of a hand, arm, foot, leg, chin, or lips. In Parkinson's disease, this usually happens while the limb is at rest, but sometimes it happens also with movement.
- **Bradykinesia:** Unusually slow movement of the limbs or the entire body.
- **Rigidity:** Stiffness of the muscles in the hand, arm, foot, leg, or trunk and neck.
- **Postural Instability:** Wobbly or unbalanced standing or walking.

Although physical symptoms are the first indications of the disease, many people with Parkinson's also experience behavioral changes, such as fatigue, apathy, depression, anxiety, and sleep problems. These behavioral symptoms are explored in more detail in Chapter 4.

> **Progression** of Parkinson's disease varies from person to person, but it may be slow and, in some cases, may never lead to significant impairment.

Medication can be very effective in treating the symptoms of Parkinson's disease. There are medications that encourage the production of dopamine in the brain or supply the brain with a substitute for dopamine. Other medications help the brain make better use of its remaining dopamine-producing capacity. Yet other medications may suppress naturally occurring chemicals that work against dopamine. All these medications help reduce shakiness, slowness, stiffness, and other symptoms in most patients. Other medications can be used to reduce the nonmotor symptoms; such medications can be memory-enhancing medications; antidepressants; and medications to help prevent low blood pressure, help with sleep, or help with bladder control. All these medication options are reviewed in Chapter 7.

> Many famous people found **inspiration and new meaning** in their lives after they were diagnosed with Parkinson's disease.

In addition to medication, certain types of therapies can help alleviate parkinsonian symptoms. Physical, occupational, and speech therapies may lead to surprising improvement of the physical symptoms, although brain surgery may be necessary when symptom control becomes unpredictable. For many people, exercise also helps reduce the symptoms associated with the disease. We discuss these treatments in Chapters 8, 9, and 10.

You Are Not Alone

When people with Parkinson's get together and share their stories, they quickly learn about the variety of ways people are affected by the illness. Many people also benefit from telling others about their experience, hearing others' experiences, and learning ways to live with the disease.

Several famous Americans have been diagnosed with Parkinson's disease, including boxer Muhammad Ali and former Attorney General Janet Reno, Michael J. Fox, Neil Diamond, Alan Alda, and many others. Each one of these inspiring people has shown that it is possible to live a fulfilling life with Parkinson's disease. In their individual ways and in their separate fields, they have made plain that life after the diagnosis of Parkinson's can be both purpose filled and rewarding.

About This Book and How to Use It

In this book, we focus on Parkinson's disease itself, clarify some misunderstandings, describe the symptoms that may occur in different stages of the disease, explore possible causes, describe how the disease is diagnosed, and discuss what can be done to treat the symptoms. We also discuss complications of the various treatments, suggest steps you can take to improve your prognosis, write about ongoing research, explore new treatment options, and suggest ways for you to continue to live a productive and rewarding life.

It has been our experience, and that of the many other physicians and healthcare professionals who treat Parkinson's disease, that one of the most important factors for successful disease management is informed patients and care partners. In the modern approach to chronic disease management, the patient is placed at the center of the team. In the team approach, the person with Parkinson's remains in charge of his or her care. The doctor and the other healthcare professionals will assess the person with Parkinson's and provide the necessary information about treatment options, so that the person with Parkinson's will be able to make the right decisions about his or her care. The team members will help out in this decision-making process through education and will try to empower the person with Parkinson's and their care partner in ways that will improve his or her long-term outlook. This model calls for patient-centered **multidisciplinary care** and interdisciplinary disease management.

Elements of Successful Disease Management

- Informed patient (and care partner or family)
- Multidisciplinary team of healthcare professionals
- Communication
- Respect for patient's priorities and wishes

Patient centered means what was just described. *Multidisciplinary* means that healthcare professionals from many fields (e.g., physical, occupational, and speech therapists; nurses; psychologists; and **exercise physiologists**) may need to provide their expert assessments and specialized treatments at various stages of the disease. *Interdisciplinary* means that all these healthcare professionals, including the doctor, need to communicate, consult with each other, and act as a team, with the aim of addressing the patient's healthcare needs and concerns while also paying attention to his or her wishes and expectations.

While knowing more about the disease is important, available information can be overwhelming. Make your **learning decisions**—that is, your decisions about what (and what not) to learn—based on your personal preferences and needs and understand that you may wish to learn smaller amounts of information at a time.

In the first few chapters of this book (Chapters 2 through 6), we try to explain the nature of the disease in terms of its symptoms, possible underlying causes, the anatomical and chemical changes that occur in the nervous system of persons living with the disease, and the various challenges patients have to face as the disease progresses. We cannot stress enough, however, how different the disease is from individual to individual. Therefore, it should not be thought that everything in this book applies to everyone who lives with Parkinson's.

In the second part of the book (Chapters 7 through 10), we address ways to manage the symptoms of the disease, including medications, exercise, therapies, surgical treatments, and lifestyle changes that may help address the challenges of living with Parkinson's. This is followed by chapters dedicated to the role of research, planning for the future, how the care partner or the patient's family can be part of the disease management strategy, and how to become involved in advocating for the Parkinson's community (Chapters 11 through 14). Finally, we include a glossary of technical terms at the end of the book.

We thought that real people's stories could help others understand their own challenges better and help them develop their own strategies for dealing with the disease. Therefore, throughout the book we have included real-life stories. In most instances, names, story details, and circumstances have been altered to conceal the person's identity.

Sometimes people want straightforward answers to very specific, frequently asked questions. We have sprinkled such "pearls of wisdom" from experts in the field in the form of Ask the Experts text boxes for quick reference.

This book cannot be either very detailed or all-encompassing. It is meant to be used as a guide. The best adviser for an individual with Parkinson's disease will be a doctor—the quarterback of her or his "team."

CHAPTER 2

What Is It? Why Me?

In this chapter, you will learn about

- Changes that happen in the brain of people with Parkinson's disease
- Theories about what causes Parkinson's disease
- Stages of Parkinson's disease
- What can be done about Parkinson's disease

"So slight and nearly imperceptible are the first inroads of this malady, and so extremely slow is its progress, that it rarely happens, that the patient can form any recollection of the precise period of its commencement." That's how James Parkinson described the beginning of the disease in his book *An Essay on the Shaking Palsy*. Parkinson wasn't the first person to notice symptoms associated with "the shaking palsy." Ancient Chinese manuscripts and medieval texts described people having the characteristic symptoms of the disease, such as tremors, slow movements, shuffling, and stooping. But, it's quite possible that not many people had the condition in those days. Most people living with Parkinson's disease are older than 60, and until the past century or so, people lived much shorter lives. Moreover, it was much easier to attribute Parkinson's symptoms to aging.

From a functional standpoint, Parkinson's disease is considered a **hypokinetic** disorder. **Hypo-** is a Greek term meaning "under," while **kinesis** means "motion." Being hypokinetic simply means that people with Parkinson's disease lack range and speed of motion in their movements. To many readers, this might not seem correct.

After all, the symptom that most people associate with Parkinson's is tremor, which is an excess of motion. Although tremor is the most visible symptom of the disease, the central symptom of Parkinson's is a slowing of movements and a stiffening of the muscles like that seen in the case of Count de Lordat (discussed in this chapter's Is There Help? section).

What Is It?

Parkinson's disease is a neurodegenerative disorder. In neurodegenerative diseases, neurons (nerve cells) die sooner than normal, both inside and outside the brain; most damage, however, occurs inside the brain. Humans are born with a specific number of neurons. As we age, many of these cells die a natural death. However, we are born with hundreds of billions of neurons in our brains, and, under normal conditions, we have plenty of "extra" nerve cells to keep the body and mind working well despite the losses. Unlike other cells, nerve cells do not reproduce to generate new nerve cells when something goes wrong. If a person loses part of the liver, the remaining liver cells will divide and multiply to produce new liver cells to replace some of the liver tissue that was lost. Another example is blood: Blood cells are constantly produced by the bone marrow throughout our lives. However, when neurons die, the remaining ones can't multiply to produce new neurons. In neurodegenerative diseases, certain types of neurons die at a much faster rate than normal "wear and tear" and are not replaced.

As discussed in Chapter 1, the neurons that are affected early in the course of Parkinson's disease are the dopaminergic neurons that live in a part of the brainstem called the substantia nigra, which is Latin for "black substance." The reason this part of the brain is called black substance is that it looks black in normal brains (as seen on the left in Figure 2.1). In Parkinson's disease, however, the substantia nigra turns pale (as seen on the right in Figure 2.1). The dopaminergic

FIGURE 2.1 Substantia nigra from a normal brain (left) and that of a Parkinson's patient (right).

neurons of the substantia nigra help regulate motion; they make our physical movements smooth and accurate, not only so that with practice a ballet dancer can perform beautiful pirouettes and a talented golfer can sink a difficult putt, but also so that one's handwriting can be smooth and legible. Dopaminergic neurons help accomplish that by fine-tuning muscle tone and closely regulating the speed of motion. When too many of these neurons die, a person's everyday motions—such as walking, talking, swallowing, and writing—are affected. Because of the imbalance of muscle tone, tremors may also appear. It is estimated that by the time a person develops the symptoms of Parkinson's, she or he has already lost about 75–80 percent of the dopaminergic neurons in the substantia nigra.

These dopaminergic neurons use dopamine to communicate messages to a part of the brain called the **striatum**. The striatum plays a pivotal role in managing movement. Once a person decides to move an arm or leg, the motor centers of the brain notify the striatum, whose job is to adjust the tone of the various muscles that are involved in the movement. The striatum also determines the force with which these muscles need to contract and the speed and order with which the muscles will have to be activated so that the movement is executed smoothly and with precision. For the striatum to achieve all this, it collects information from all over the body—including the muscles, joints, eyes, and ears—about the locations of arms, legs, hands, and feet and their relation to the space and objects surrounding us. Even simple tasks require the brain to make an amazing number of calculations and communications between the brain and the body to be nearly instantaneous. Washing a bowl in a sink of bubbly water requires the brain and body working together to calculate water temperature; to pick up a sponge, scrub, and rinse; to examine the cleanliness of the bowl; to put the bowl on a drying rack; and to take care of many other details of the task that we don't even think about.

While all of this is taking place, the substantia nigra neurons use dopamine to help "fine-tune" the neurons that live in the striatum by adjusting their level of excitability (receptiveness to new information). The nerve fibers of the dopamine neurons in the substantia nigra accomplish this function by delivering small amounts of dopamine through their connections, called synapses, to the neurons of the striatum. Dopamine exerts a "push" action on some nerve cells and a "pull" action on others, and this push-pull action helps fine-tune the striatum neurons. This fine-tuning is lost when the dopamine neurons of the substantia nigra degenerate, as is the case in Parkinson's disease. A person's movements then become less smooth, stiffer (rigidity), and slower (bradykinesia), and the movements appear more hesitant and deliberate, as if "the brakes are on" throughout any type of voluntary movement.

Although the most visible symptoms of Parkinson's occur when the dopaminergic neurons of substantia nigra are affected by the disease process, neurons in other parts of the brain and the **autonomic nervous system** (which controls body functions that a person doesn't have to think about, e.g., heartbeat, sweating, and the movements of the stomach and intestines) will also be involved in time. As a result, people living with Parkinson's may often experience additional symptoms that are not related to the amount of dopamine in their brain; therefore, such symptoms may not respond to dopamine-enhancing drugs. In our current understanding, Parkinson's is a disease that affects many parts of the nervous system, so the treatments we use, and ultimately a cure for the disease, will have to look past the improved function or preservation of the dopaminergic neurons alone.

What Causes Parkinson's Disease?

Lewy Bodies

We do not know exactly what kills neurons in Parkinson's disease. However, using a microscope, if we look at the substantia nigra of a brain affected with Parkinson's, we see an accumulation of material inside the bodies of those neurons that have been affected by the disease process. This accumulated material is called **Lewy bodies** and consists of clogged clumps of damaged proteins (see Figure 2.2). One of the main damaged proteins that accumulate in Lewy bodies is **α-synuclein**. This fact is important because some of the genetic forms of Parkinson's disease involve an abnormal **gene** that results in production of an abnormal form of α-synuclein. The abnormally formed α-synuclein molecules have a greater tendency to clump together and form Lewy bodies. Proteins are long molecules that are supposed to have a normal three-dimensional structure to be functional. A good analogy would be a coiled telephone cord. In the normal state, it has a nice spring and elasticity to it; however, if it is twisted the wrong way, it bundles up and can no longer expand properly, losing its elasticity and function. Similarly, if the α-synuclein molecule gets misfolded (because of either an error in its genetic blueprint or other reasons, some of which we discuss further in this chapter), it can lose its proper function, and, what's more important, it may form aggregates (clumps) inside the neurons. Scientists have now confirmed that the abnormally folded α-synuclein is poisonous to the neurons in which it aggregates. The same abnormally folded α-synuclein is found in Lewy bodies in the neurons of people with Parkinson's even without the

FIGURE 2.2 Interior of a dopaminergic neuron from the substantia nigra of a patient with Parkinson's. The round object by the arrow is a Lewy body.

abnormal α-synuclein gene. Therefore, it is now believed that many possible factors, both genetic and environmental or combinations of genetic and environmental factors, may lead to the production and aggregation of abnormally formed, toxic α-synuclein in Lewy bodies. What's more, there are indications that the poisonous molecule may spread from one neuron to the next, thereby spreading the disease throughout the nervous system. As new studies help us understand this process better, researchers are beginning to identify new opportunities for therapies that may stop disease progression. But, more on that further in this chapter.

Another protein seen in the Lewy bodies is called **ubiquitin**. This fact is also important because, in some other **hereditary** forms of Parkinson's, an abnormal gene causes ubiquitin to function abnormally. Ubiquitin's role has to do with the breakup and elimination of damaged and aged proteins inside neurons. One of the theories regarding why substantia nigra neurons die in Parkinson's disease hypothesizes that the inability to process old and damaged proteins leads to their accumulation inside the neuron and its eventual demise due to their toxic effects.

Ask the Experts: What Is a Lewy Body?

Dr. Martha Nance says, "The Lewy body is a black spot that the pathologist can see inside the damaged nerve cells in the brain of a person with Parkinson's disease or the related condition **Lewy body disease**. These blobs of protein are named after Dr. Frederick Lewy, the neurologist who discovered them. Lewy bodies are seen in a small number of cells early in Parkinson's disease but are more widespread throughout the brain in the later stages of the disease. People with Lewy body disease have more Lewy bodies throughout the brain early in the course of their disease which reflects that this condition includes not only a Parkinson's-like movement disorder but also cognitive changes (**dementia**) and hallucinations at the onset of the disease.

"Scientists are currently trying to determine whether Lewy bodies cause damage to nerve cells or whether they reflect the cells' best efforts to clean up the mess. There is increasing evidence that the Lewy body contains "worn-out" proteins that should be handled by the cell's recycling system (called the **proteasome**). In Parkinson's disease, it seems that the proteasome gets overwhelmed and can't keep up, and protein 'trash' collects inside the cell. The Lewy body may represent the cell's attempt to 'sweep the trash into the corner' so that the cell can keep functioning.

"Two of the genes that have been implicated in Parkinson's disease are important in the recycling pathway. **Parkin** is a protein that is responsible for 'tagging' proteins to be moved to the proteasome for recycling. A mutation in the parkin gene, then, interferes with the tagging and recycling process and allows the protein trash to accumulate in the cells. α-Synuclein is the main protein found in the Lewy body. Mutations in the gene for α-synuclein cause hereditary Parkinson's disease. A mutation in the α-synuclein gene leads *to the production of a faulty α-synuclein protein, which ends up in the 'trash pile' sooner than a normal α-synuclein protein.*

"In addition, at least in the test tube, exposure to herbicides and heavy metals such as manganese and aluminum increases the tendency of α-synuclein to form protein clumps. Perhaps— nobody knows this for sure—this has something to do with the increased risk of Parkinson's disease in welders and farmers.

"Why some people develop Lewy bodies in a small area of the brain (Parkinson's disease) while others seem to have a much broader distribution of Lewy bodies even early in their disease course (Lewy body disease) is entirely unknown."

Other Theories About the Cause of Parkinson's Disease

There are many more theories about what causes Parkinson's disease, and in the following paragraphs, we discuss some prominent examples. One theory centers on oxidative stress. Like other cells in our body, neurons use oxygen to produce energy to survive and function properly. The chemical reactions that happen inside cells to extract energy from oxygen molecules produce by-products called **free radicals**, which can damage nerve cells. Neurons normally have the ability to neutralize free radicals and so protect themselves from damage. **Antioxidants** (e.g., vitamins C and E) are chemicals that boost this neutralizing ability of cells. In fact, oxidation—the chemical process through which energy is produced from oxygen—is considered an important cause of aging. That is why antioxidants are very popular not only as nutritional supplements for persons with neurodegenerative diseases but also as components of products touted as antiaging remedies. In the context of Parkinson's disease, the theory of oxidative stress postulates that there is a breakdown in the ability of the dopaminergic neurons to process an excess amount of toxic free radicals, which leads to their death.

Another popular theory centers on mitochondrial dysfunction. **Mitochondria** are small particles inside the neurons that capture energy from oxygen molecules so that it can be used for the cell's metabolic processes (the constant renewal of the cell's components). These processes are necessary for the ongoing function and survival of the neuron. Many studies have shown that there is some degree of mitochondrial dysfunction in neurons and other cells of people with Parkinson's disease. In fact, mitochondrial dysfunction leads to an increase of oxidative stress, which was discussed in the previous paragraph. So it's possible that the demise of the substantia nigra neurons results from the reduced ability of mitochondria to use oxygen efficiently. This has led to further speculation that some nutritional supplements that may improve mitochondrial function may also help slow the progression of Parkinson's. One such supplement, coenzyme Q10, had shown promise for slowing the disease's progression in a few early small studies. However, a very large study funded by the National Institutes of Health could not confirm the usefulness of this supplement in slowing Parkinson's progression.

Processing of iron in the striatum and the substantia nigra can also produce excessive free radicals inside the dopaminergic neurons and thereby contribute to their early demise. Modern research techniques involving the use of **magnetic resonance imaging (MRI)** machines with very powerful magnets have provided measurements indicating that, at least in some forms of Parkinson's, increased iron content is present in the striatum and the substantia nigra. Such measurements have supported a role for iron in the genesis of Parkinson's disease, but a lot more research is needed before we fully understand the importance of such a connection.

Inflammation in the brain has also been considered as a cause for the loss of dopaminergic neurons. Some infectious diseases, including lethargic encephalitis, West Nile encephalitis, and mycoplasma pneumonia, can cause inflammation in the brain that may damage neurons, including those in the substantia nigra. Physicians have a long tradition of trying anti-inflammatory medications as treatments for neurodegenerative diseases. A group of scientists from the University of Washington published a critical review of 11 studies on the relationship between the use of anti-inflammatories and the risk for developing Parkinson's disease. The group concluded that these studies collectively supported the notion that regular use of these drugs was associated with a slightly lower probability of developing Parkinson's disease. A word of caution: Such "observational" studies are usually able to demonstrate associations; however, they cannot establish a cause-and-effect relationship. This means that it does not necessarily follow from these studies that taking anti-inflammatories is a good thing for people with Parkinson's or people who are at risk of getting the disease. Such studies do, however, lend support to the idea that inflammation may be one of the mechanisms that cause Parkinson's disease.

This list of possible explanations of neuronal damage in Parkinson's disease is by no means inclusive. New theories are published frequently in medical journals and usually have considerable scientific merit. To test such theories, scientists have developed several animal models of Parkinson's disease—that is, procedures that produce symptoms like those of Parkinson's in animals. Unfortunately, none of the models fully replicates how Parkinson's develops in people. Any conclusions drawn from such laboratory studies continue to be hypothetical and need to be examined further to see whether they apply to people as well as to rats or monkeys.

> Doctors use the **Hoehn and Yahr scale** to report the degree of disease progression and the **Unified Parkinson's Disease Rating Scale** (UPDRS) to describe the severity of the symptoms and signs of Parkinson's.

What Are the Stages of the Disease?

All the theories discussed so far are centered on the substantia nigra, which is in the brainstem. New research shows that the disease process affects other parts of the brain even before it reaches the substantia nigra. This discovery has led scientists to examine the progress of the disease by conducting autopsies to track the pathologic staging of Parkinson's disease. By looking at the autopsied brain of patients with Parkinson's, scientists can judge the extent of the disease from the distribution of the Lewy bodies. Professor Heiko Braak of the Johann Wolfgang Goethe University in Frankfurt, Germany, developed a way of staging the disease based on the extent of pathologic changes in the brain of deceased people with Parkinson's.

How do the Lewy bodies and, therefore, the disease progress through the brain? In 2008, two groups of scientists, one from the United States and one from Sweden, reported their findings from autopsies of three people with Parkinson's who had received fetal cell transplants into their brains in an effort to replace their dying dopaminergic neurons. The grafts had survived, and the patients lived for more than 10 years, but when scientists examined their brains after they had died, they found that the grafted cells had been afflicted with Lewy bodies. This was the first indication that somehow the disease spreads from one neuron to the next.

Knowing that many people with Parkinson's have had either loss of smell or constipation for many years before any kind of **motor symptoms** became visible, scientists started questioning whether the disease process starts outside the brain, in nerve endings in the nose or nerve endings in the gut. Something—maybe a chemical or a virus—triggers the misfolding of α-synuclein and the formation of Lewy bodies in these nerve endings. It's also possible that this process may be triggered only in people who have a certain genetic sensitivity to the particular chemical or virus. Once the process is started, it takes on a life of its own and continues to progress. The misformed α-synuclein slowly makes its way from one neuron to the next, all the way into the brain and finally to the substantia nigra; once sufficient damage to the substantia nigra has occurred, the motor symptoms of Parkinson's arise. If that proves indeed to be the case, there may be a long stage of the disease that lasts many years, even decades, before the tremors, rigidity, or bradykinesia show up for the first time. Doctors and scientists have been using the term *premanifest Parkinson's disease* when they talk about this early "silent" stage of the Parkinson's disease process.

When determining the disease stage based on clinical symptoms and findings, doctors do not have the benefit of examining the patient's brain under the microscope. In 1967, Drs. Margaret Hoehn and Melvin Yahr developed a staging system for Parkinson's disease based on motor symptoms. This five-stage measurement tool gives physicians and patients a rough idea of the progress of the disease. Here's a brief description of the Hoehn and Yahr stages of Parkinson's disease:

- **Stage** 1: People with Parkinson's disease who have symptoms only on one side of the body, such as a tremor or some rigidity and slowness of movement in one arm or leg (or both, if on the same side of the body).
- **Stage 2:** Symptoms appear on both sides of the body or in the midline of the body, including decreased facial expression, drooling, stooping, or shuffling while walking. However, there are no problems with balance. The first two stages are considered early or mild.
- **Stage 3:** As soon as a person begins having trouble with balance, she or he has crossed into Stage 3. In this stage, patients don't need help walking or getting up from a sitting position, but their body movements are becoming increasingly slow. The disease is now considered to be mild to moderate.
- **Stage 4:** A person with Parkinson's can no longer be completely independent. Symptoms, including disabling slowness of movement and stiffness, are moderate to severe. The disease's impact on balance and walking is so great that the person usually needs help—from another person or an assistive device—to walk. However, the person is still able to get up from bed or from a chair without help.

- **Stage 5:** Once a person with Parkinson's is unable to get up from a bed or chair without help, they have crossed into Stage 5. The person requires help or even nursing care for the majority of daily activities.

Thanks to **levodopa** (also called **L-dopa**)—our most effective drug to treat the symptoms of Parkinson's disease—determining how far the disease has progressed has become more complex. For example, when a patient is taking medications, he or she may qualify for a Stage 2 rating, but when the medications don't work, the same person may function only at the level of Stage 4.

Neurologists also use a standardized scoring system to rate the severity (as opposed to the stage) of the motor symptoms of Parkinson's disease. The UPDRS system was developed in the 1980s and was revised in 2008 by the International Parkinson and Movement Disorder Society, an association of neurologists specializing in the treatment of Parkinson's disease and other movement disorders. The UPDRS consists of a number of questions and an examination. The answers to the questions and the severity of the signs of the disease found during the examination are rated, for the most part, on a scale of 0–4. The sum of these ratings is the UPDRS score. This is a useful way for physicians to measure a patient's progress from visit to visit and to assess when medications work or don't work. However, the scale has limitations for comparing the severity of the illness of different patients. The same score in two patients may actually be associated with different degrees of severity and different types of symptoms and impairment.

Some of the shortcomings of the UPDRS were addressed and corrected in 2008, when a team of movement disorders specialists were tasked by the International Parkinson and Movement Disorder Society to develop and test an updated version of the UPDRS. This scale, called the MDS-UPDRS (MDS for Movement Disorder Society), is more detailed and collects information about many other areas and experiences of daily living that are affected in the day-to-day lives of people with Parkinson's.

We know today that the cardinal symptoms are only a "slice of the pie" that's called Parkinson's disease. As people living with Parkinson's have always known and doctors who treat them have come to realize in the past couple of decades, the disease affects people's lives in many nonvisible ways. Constipation, poor sleep, lightheadedness, fatigue, depression and anxiety, hallucinations, and even dementia may often have a more dramatic effect on people's lives than tremor and rigidity. Again, through international collaboration, Parkinson's doctors have created a Non-Motor Symptoms Scale for Parkinson's disease (NMSS for short). Doctors will also often use different scales to measure the severity of the symptoms, such as scales to assess **cognition**, depressive symptoms, anxiety, and so on.

> **Age, genetics, and environmental exposures** may all contribute to a person's risk of developing Parkinson's disease.

Who Gets the Disease? Why Me?

When diagnosed with an illness, one of the first questions people ask is straightforward: "Why me?" For Parkinson's disease, as with most diseases affecting the brain, the answer is not simple. Age, genetics, and exposure to certain environmental conditions may be risk factors in the development of Parkinson's disease, but no single thing is known to be its cause. In the next few paragraphs, we explore risk factors that may contribute to a person developing Parkinson's disease.

Age is one of the leading factors associated with the risk of developing Parkinson's. Older people are more likely to have the disease than the young. Close to 1.5 million people in the United States are currently living with Parkinson's disease, and approximately 50,000 Americans alone are diagnosed with the disease every year;

most of them are over the age of 60. However, people as young as 20 or older than 100 may develop Parkinson's. The aging of the baby boomer generation is expected to boost the number of people living with Parkinson's disease, which is the second most common neurodegenerative disease after Alzheimer's disease. Statistics suggest that Parkinson's disease strikes men slightly more often than women (approximately six men get Parkinson's for every four women who are diagnosed with the disease), and that it is slightly more frequent among whites than among Africans, Asians, and Native Americans.

Another risk factor is genetics. To determine if Parkinson's disease runs in families, researchers have conducted many large studies of hundreds of people with and without Parkinson's disease. They found that if you don't have a relative with Parkinson's disease, your lifetime risk for the disease is about 2 percent. If you have a relative with Parkinson's disease, your lifetime risk for the disease is about 4 percent. Between 5 and 15 percent of people with Parkinson's are likely to have inherited the disease itself or the tendency to develop it. With the development of the science of genetics in recent decades, variants of a number of genes have been identified that cause Parkinson's disease; this has contributed greatly to our understanding of the mechanisms of the disease. For most of our genes, we inherit two copies, one from our father and one from our mother. Some of these inherited genes are *dominant,* which means that we need only one abnormal copy to get the disease. With dominant genes, then, one of the parents must have the abnormal gene—and therefore the disease—for a child also to get it. Other genes are *recessive.* Recessive genes require a person to have two abnormal copies to get the disease: one from the father and one from the mother. In this case, the person's parents both carry the abnormal gene but neither one may actually have Parkinson's disease since each may have only one copy of the abnormal gene.

Another category of genes that scientists are looking at with great interest is *susceptibility* genes. A person with a susceptibility gene may have a higher risk of getting Parkinson's than those without. Yet most people with the gene will still not get Parkinson's. Scientists have been finding more and more evidence of interactions between genes and environmental factors, and we may someday find out that there are certain combinations of influences from the environment that can trigger the disease only in people with the corresponding combination of susceptibility genes.

Some of the most discussed genes associated with Parkinson's disease are the α-synuclein gene (also called *SNCA*), the dardarin gene (or *LRRK2*), the parkin gene (*PRKN*), and the glucocerebrosidase gene (*GBA1*). Some of the gene mutations that are particularly associated with heightened risk for the disease are much more frequently encountered among people who have a particular ethnic background. One example is the *GBA1* gene, which is very frequently seen among people of Ashkenazi Jewish ancestry with Parkinson's. People who contract Parkinson's at a younger age are more likely to have a genetic abnormality at the root of their disease. Indications are that there may be some differences in the outlook of people with Parkinson's who carry a particular gene mutation compared to those without. It is also possible that certain treatments may work better for some people than others, depending on their harboring a gene mutation. It is also possible that in the future, knowledge of a person's genetic background may be useful in deciding which treatments may be best for the particular person. This way of informing treatment based on a person's genetics is called **personalized medicine**.

Ask the Experts: Is Parkinson's Disease Hereditary?

*Dr. Martha Nance says, "For two centuries, the prevailing view among researchers has been that Parkinson's disease is (usually) not hereditary. We have known for many years that about 15–20 percent of people living with Parkinson's disease also have relatives with the ailment. But that observation alone doesn't prove the illness is hereditary, as relatives also tend to live in similar environments. In recent years, studies of the human **genome** have* *begun to identify genes and genetic variants that can be associated with or, in rare cases, cause Parkinson's disease. However, the presence of Parkinson's disease–associated genetic variants still only increases the lifetime risk of contracting the disease from 2–2.4 percent. The α-synuclein (SNCA), tau (MAPT), and leucine rich repeat kinase (LRRK2) genes have most convincingly been associated with an increased risk for Parkinson's disease.*

"Mutations that can outright cause Parkinson's disease are rare but have been reported in a number of genes, including SNCA, PRKN, UCHL1, DJ1, PINK1, GBA1, and LRRK2. Specific mutations in these genes can cause multiple people in the same family to get Parkinson's disease. Although it is uncommon for a person with Parkinson's disease to have a mutation in one or another of these genes (I have treated one patient who had a SNCA mutation in over 25 years of Parkinson's disease care), the knowledge that a single gene mutation can, in itself, cause Parkinson's disease has significantly helped to guide research in Parkinson's disease. So, although the majority of people with Parkinson's disease do not have an identifiable, specific, disease-causing gene mutation and work continues to identify environmental or age-related factors that cause the disease, we will learn more in the coming years about how a person's underlying genetic makeup influences the response to environmental stresses and ultimately leads to Parkinson's disease."

But what then about the role of our environment? How about chemicals in the air, the water, the food we eat? Studies have shown that people with long-term exposure to some organic solvents, pesticides, and herbicides are at higher risk of developing Parkinson's disease. People who live in rural areas and drink well water most of their lives or who live near wood pulp–processing plants are also at higher risk of contracting Parkinson's. However, most people with Parkinson's disease have never had exposure to these environmental conditions, and most people who were exposed don't get Parkinson's.

In the 1980s, Dr. William Langston observed that some drug users in the San Francisco Bay Area developed a rapidly progressing form of parkinsonism. It took some fascinating medical detective work (which Dr. Langston described in his book *The Case of the Frozen Addicts*) to figure out that the culprit was a chemical called MPTP that was a by-product in the preparation of certain illegal drugs in "kitchen labs." MPTP acts as a neurotoxin and has a particular affinity for the dopamine neurons of the substantia nigra. It quickly kills a large number of these neurons, causing a condition very similar to Parkinson's disease. However, the difference is that MPTP parkinsonism is not a progressive illness like Parkinson's disease, and, although it causes many similar symptoms, it does not necessarily represent the same mechanisms that are at work in Parkinson's.

The discovery of MPTP triggered more studies of chemicals with chemical structures similar to MPTP. Some of these chemicals are used as herbicides and pesticides. One of them called paraquat has been studied extensively and has been found to increase the risk of getting Parkinson's about threefold. Studies have shown that people with long-term exposure to several other organic solvents, pesticides, and herbicides are at higher risk of developing Parkinson's disease. People who live in rural areas and drink well water most of their lives or who live near wood pulp–processing plants are also at higher risk of contracting Parkinson's. However, most people with Parkinson's disease never had exposure to these environmental conditions, and the vast majority of people who were exposed don't get Parkinson's.

> Exposure to **paraquat**, a pesticide, triples the risk of getting Parkinson's disease.

Some occupations also have been associated with a higher risk of Parkinson's disease, including farming, teaching, anesthesiology, and welding (although there are some conflicting studies on this last one). There are several theories about why people in these occupations are vulnerable to Parkinson's disease. For example, manganese poisoning, which can cause symptoms similar to Parkinson's, has been offered as a possible explanation for welders' raised risk, as has pesticide exposure for that of farmers. However, there is no definitive explanation for any of these occupational associations.

Researchers have also studied whether certain infections or severe head injuries can make a person more likely to contract Parkinson's disease. No particular infection has been consistently associated with Parkinson's, although a number of brain infections can cause illnesses that resemble Parkinson's disease. The most notable infection causing signs similar to Parkinson's disease is lethargic encephalitis, also known as the sleeping sickness. Likewise, studies examining a possible connection between head injuries and Parkinson's disease have proved inconclusive. In a very interesting study, Dr. Samuel Goldman reported that some people who have one particular variant of the α-synuclein gene (the abnormal variants of which can cause a hereditary form of Parkinson's) have a higher risk for developing Parkinson's after head injuries than people who do not possess that variant.

But what about any "protective" influences in the environment? Are there any chemicals or environmental exposures that protect people from getting Parkinson's? The answer is that we do not know. It has been established, for example, that people who smoke and people who consume a lot of caffeine have a somewhat lower risk of developing Parkinson's. Does that mean that these chemicals may protect against Parkinson's? Most likely the answer is no. It appears that dopamine is very much involved in the development of habits and addictive behaviors, and it is likely that the reduced dopamine levels in the parkinsonian brain may make people destined to develop Parkinson's less susceptible to habits such as smoking and drinking too much coffee. There may also be common genetic factors that make people more likely to start smoking but at the same time less likely to develop Parkinson's disease. There is too much we do not fully understand about such interactions to draw any valid conclusions. Some clinical trials have been conducted to see whether nicotine or caffeine slow down disease progression in people with Parkinson's, but they have been unsuccessful.

> The "**loaded gun**" **theory** of the cause of Parkinson's disease postulates that a person's genetic makeup loads the gun but that some environmental factor is necessary to "pull the trigger."

Is There Help?

Count de Lordat was a "handsome, middle-sized, sanguine man, of cheerful disposition, and an active mind." Nearly 4 years after he first developed symptoms of the disease, James Parkinson described the man this way: "He still walked alone with a cane, from one room to the other, but with great difficulty, and in a tottering manner; his left hand and arm were much reduced, and would hardly perform any motion; the right was somewhat benumbed, and he could scarcely lift it up to his head; his saliva was continually trickling out of his mouth, and he had neither the power of retaining it, nor of spitting it out freely." Fortunately, modern medicine has considerably improved the lives of people with Parkinson's, and the count would have done much better today.

Insights on how to treat Parkinson's disease with medications didn't emerge until the mid-twentieth century, when physicians noticed that patients with schizophrenia on antipsychotic drugs began developing symptoms of Parkinson's disease. So, researchers began examining possible relationships between the antipsychotic drugs and the cause of Parkinson's disease. These scientists discovered that the antipsychotic drugs deprived the brain of the effects of dopamine. Pathologists already knew that the substantia nigra appeared very pale in the brain of people who had died of Parkinson's disease, in contrast to normal brains, where it had an intense blue-black hue. As it turns out, the neurons of the substantia nigra produce dopamine, and dopamine turns black when it's packaged for storage inside these cells. Putting two and two together, scientists realized that the loss of dopamine in the brainstem was the cause of the symptoms of Parkinson's disease.

So, why not just give patients with Parkinson's dopamine pills to replace the loss of dopamine in the brain? Doctors tried that, but there was a problem. Without a healthy brain, the body can't function, so the brain has a kind of protective shield called the **blood-brain barrier**. This barrier is a system of specialized cells and processes designed to keep the brain safe from toxins and infections. The blood-brain barrier is therefore a very good thing, but it does make it trickier for doctors to help patients with brain disorders like Parkinson's disease because dopamine cannot cross it.

In 1968, Dr. George C. Cotzias published a scientific article in the *New England Journal of Medicine* titled "Levodopa for Parkinsonism." Based on laboratory research, Cotzias suggested treating people with Parkinson's with high doses of levodopa because levodopa crosses the blood-brain barrier and the neurons can convert levodopa into dopamine. Although doctors had already tried this approach without success, Dr. Cotzias used the drug at much higher dosages than the ones that had been previously tried. Once levodopa crosses the blood-brain barrier and is inside the brain, it reaches the brainstem and gets transformed into dopamine, temporarily enabling people with Parkinson's to regain control and fluidity of their movements while also reducing tremor and muscle stiffness.

Awakenings, a 1990 film starring Robin Williams and Robert De Niro, was based on real patient stories taken from a book in which Dr. Oliver Sacks described the impact of levodopa on patients who had had Parkinson's symptoms for many years.

The introduction of levodopa to treat Parkinson's disease in 1968 generated optimism among neurologists that there really was an effective treatment for Parkinson's disease. Unfortunately, levodopa doesn't cure Parkinson's; it merely treats its symptoms, causing temporary relief from the long-term, debilitating effects of the illness. As the disease progresses, damage spreads to other neurons that are *not* dependent on dopamine for their function. When this happens, people with Parkinson's may develop symptoms that are not improved by enhancing the dopamine content of the brain. Nonetheless, researchers such as Dr. Ryan Uitti of the Mayo Clinic in Jacksonville, Florida, have demonstrated that the introduction of levodopa has dramatically increased the life span of people living with Parkinson's. It comes as no surprise that levodopa is considered one of the greatest breakthroughs in medical therapeutics in the twentieth century.

In the 1970s and 1980s, research on medication for Parkinson's focused on optimizing the use of levodopa and minimizing the drug's side effects. The resulting advances allowed people to live fuller, longer lives, but they also presented a challenge. As people with Parkinson's disease lived longer, the disease began affecting parts of the brain that were spared in earlier stages. Early in its course, Parkinson's disease affects how well people can walk, talk, write, and perform other daily activities. Later in the disease, however, it can also affect thinking and cause unexplained falling, confusion, or fainting, which are symptoms that not only do not respond to additional dopamine but also may, in fact, get worse from it.

The Outlook for People with Parkinson's

The prognosis of Parkinson's disease has changed considerably over the years. Before the advent of levodopa and other effective treatments for the motor symptoms of Parkinson's disease, the average survival after diagnosis was approximately 5 years. (This means that about 50 percent of people diagnosed with Parkinson's disease died within

5 years.) The average survival after diagnosis has since improved dramatically. Today, it is calculated that, on average, the life expectancy of a person with Parkinson's disease is approximately 18 months to 2 years less than that of people without the disease. It is not unusual for many people who have lived with Parkinson's disease for years to die "with" rather than "from" Parkinson's. However, survival varies dramatically among patients.

Some people experience a quick and aggressive form of the disease. In other people, the disease makes only slow and subtle changes to the body, so they do not experience much decline from one year to the next. About 1 in 10 people with Parkinson's has a very benign version of the disease and experiences very slow progression. It so happens that patients who have a more benign course tend to have more tremors when first diagnosed with the disease. This has led some experts to distinguish these patients as having **benign tremulous parkinsonism**. Patients with a younger age of onset have a better overall prognosis in terms of survival and the ability to retain the benefits from anti-Parkinson's medications. However, younger patients also have a greater chance of experiencing treatment complications.

Our ability to treat the motor symptoms of Parkinson's disease is better now than, say, 50 years ago, but extending the life expectancy of people with Parkinson's disease has led to some unforeseen consequences. Since people with Parkinson's disease now live longer, the disease spreads further in their brains, causing more and more symptoms for which we have not yet found very effective treatments. Researchers now believe that about one in three people with Parkinson's disease will end up developing dementia. In addition, about one in three people with Parkinson's disease will end up having to use a walker, wheelchair, or other gait-assistive device. Patients with Parkinson's disease are more likely to be admitted to a nursing home than the general population.

Over the past few years, specialists treating people with Parkinson's have become increasingly aware of these problems and have turned their attention to new research designed to address problems and symptoms that emerge in the later stages of the disease and for which no effective treatment is yet available. This line of research is almost as important as the line of research looking for a cure for the disease or for medications that may slow its progression. If researchers can find treatments that will not only prolong the life of people with Parkinson's but also eliminate problems that diminish their quality of life, then finding a cure may become less critical.

In parallel with research geared toward improving the quality of life of people with advanced Parkinson's, research efforts are increasingly focused on slowing the progression of the disease and finding a cure for it. New hope for a cure has been spurred by our increasingly detailed understanding of the processes that lead to premature neuronal death. This new information has been provided by recent advances in genetics and stem cell research. New approaches to testing new medications as possible curative agents may eliminate the need for very long, elaborate, and expensive drug trials while dramatically increasing the number of drugs that can be tested simultaneously. Cross-pollination with ideas, theories, and experimental data from research on other neurodegenerative diseases (e.g., Alzheimer's disease) or even from basic research in disciplines as diverse as chemical engineering, wearable monitoring device technology, and nanotechnology, greatly facilitated by the widespread use of the Internet, has opened new avenues to explore. There is general optimism among Parkinson's disease specialists that drugs that treat the disease itself, not just the symptoms, and even a cure may not be that far off.

CHAPTER 3

The Motor Symptoms

In this chapter, you will learn about

- The motor symptoms of Parkinson's
- How the various motor symptoms affect the functions of the body
- Motor symptoms caused by Parkinson's versus those related to the medications used to treat the disease

In 1817 (just over 200 years ago), Dr. James Parkinson first described what have become known as the classic symptoms of Parkinson's disease: tremor, rigidity (muscle stiffness), and bradykinesia (slowness of movement). To these three symptoms, modern neurologists have added the "loss of postural correcting reflexes" (balance trouble). A great many of the motor difficulties patients notice can be explained as manifestations of these four so-called cardinal symptoms. For example, **micrographia**, the small and scrawny handwriting that many people with Parkinson's have, is really a manifestation of bradykinesia. In this and the next chapter, we explore and explain common and not-so-common symptoms that people living with Parkinson's develop throughout the course of the disease.

A person with Parkinson's disease may not have all four cardinal symptoms. For example, one in four people with the disease never experiences tremor. There is only one exception to this rule: bradykinesia. According to the most accepted set of diagnostic criteria for Parkinson's disease, bradykinesia must be present or the diagnosis cannot be made with a reasonable degree of certainty. That is, a person cannot be diagnosed with Parkinson's disease unless he or she exhibits bradykinesia. By itself, however, bradykinesia is not sufficient to establish the diagnosis. One of the other three cardinal symptoms also must be present.

This list of four symptoms does not, by any means, describe the whole spectrum of motor symptoms of Parkinson's disease. Many patients may have other motor symptoms not explained by these four main symptoms, such as **dystonia**, the abnormal simultaneous contraction of muscles normally having opposing functions, or motor symptoms related to their medications, such as **dyskinesias**, which are erratic, involuntary movements of the arm, leg, trunk, or face muscles. The following sections describe and explain the various motor symptoms of the disease, including some of the more unusual ones, and discuss their potential impact on people's lives.

Tremor

Tremor is the most visible symptom of Parkinson's. For many people, whether they have the disease or not, any experience of tremor raises the worry, "Do I have Parkinson's?" The tremor has been such a fixture of the disease in people's imaginations that James Parkinson's name for it, "the shaking palsy," remains very much in use. Yet as mentioned, not everyone with Parkinson's disease gets tremors. (About 20–25 percent of people with Parkinson's never experience tremors.)

Tremor usually shows up first in one arm or leg and may even affect only a single finger. It is more likely to happen when the arm or leg is resting, then stop or subside as soon as the person moves the arm or leg. Therefore, it's often called rest or resting tremor. The arm or leg may begin shaking at times of increased stress, fear, or anger or in other emotional situations. It may appear only when the person is walking with the arm dangling at his or her side. Sometimes it may give the impression that the person is rubbing something between the thumb and pointer finger. (That's why the term *pill-rolling tremor* is sometimes used.) As time passes and the disease worsens, the tremor may be more persistent, appear even with movement of the arm or leg, spread to bigger muscles of the affected limb, or appear in other limbs as well. It generally remains most severe in the arm or leg in which it started.

Tremors have a somewhat unusual relationship with the progression of the disease and often change over time. Thus, in some people, tremor may be the main symptom at the beginning of the disease and then dissipate or even disappear as the disease worsens. In others, tremor may be very severe from the start and not respond well to medications. Interestingly, the presence of tremor early on is a good prognostic sign, which is to say that people with a tremor-predominant clinical picture tend to do better over the years than patients who have no tremor at the time of diagnosis. Drs. Margaret Hoehn and Melvin Yahr reported their study on the natural progression of Parkinson's disease in 1967, just before levodopa began to be used as a very effective treatment of the symptoms. After reviewing the cases of 802 patients, they concluded that "at least during the first ten years of the illness, parkinsonism with tremor as the initial symptom progresses more slowly than parkinsonism with other heralding symptoms." Neurologists sometimes use the term *benign tremulous parkinsonism* to describe patients who have mostly a rest tremor with few, if any, other symptoms of the disease.

> **Tremor** at the time of diagnosis may sometimes, but not always, be a sign of a more benign course.

Tremor can be difficult to treat and may be disabling. Although most Parkinson's disease medications are quite effective in controlling or even fully eliminating tremor, they don't always work. Approximately one in five people with Parkinson's may have treatment-resistant tremor, which means that the tremor cannot be fully or even partially controlled with medications.

Bradykinesia

Bradykinesia is a Greek word that means "slow movement." According to the most widely accepted diagnostic criteria for Parkinson's, if bradykinesia is not present, a diagnosis of Parkinson's disease cannot be made with certainty. Although the term implies slowness, it also refers to the size of the movements. Not only do people living with Parkinson's disease move more slowly, but also their movements are smaller. So when a neurologist examines how fast a patient can tap the pointer finger and the thumb against each other, the doctor is looking at how big those movements are as well as the speed of the movement. Many patients will make progressively smaller movements when asked to perform the task repeatedly.

> In the absence of **bradykinesia** (slow movements), a doctor cannot make the diagnosis of Parkinson's disease.

This slowing and size reduction in movements may show itself in several ways. Handwriting often becomes smaller, and it takes more time to write words. Many people also experience a loss of arm swing when walking. Other examples of bradykinesia include loss of facial expression with less blinking of the eyes (the "mask face"), slurred speech, soft voice, loss of manual dexterity, difficulty getting up from a low chair, and shuffling of steps while walking.

Bradykinesia also affects reaction time. A person with Parkinson's who trips while walking may fall because he or she isn't quick enough to recover balance. Bradykinesia may have been the cause of the tripping in the first place: persons with Parkinson's don't lift their feet high enough to clear obstacles when walking. Bradykinesia is also the reason that people with Parkinson's disease may have difficulty getting up from a low seat, getting in and out of a car, and getting in and out of bed. In the early stages, bradykinesia usually happens on either the right or left side of a person, but over time, it will spread to the other side as well.

Medications used to treat the motor symptoms of Parkinson's disease are quite effective with bradykinesia, especially in the early stages of the illness. Additionally, special exercises have been developed to address this problem. These treatments are discussed in detail in Chapters 7, 8, and 9.

Rigidity

Rigidity is the medical term for stiffness. Our muscles are never fully relaxed, but they maintain a level of muscle tone when at rest. This resting muscle tone is increased in patients with Parkinson's disease. Just like tremor and bradykinesia, this symptom is worse on one side of the body than the other. People may experience rigidity as muscle tightness, but they may also experience it as a painful, cramplike sensation in the muscles or as muscle spasms. Sometimes an achy, tired feeling may be the only indication of rigidity, and often, in the earliest stages, people with Parkinson's may be misdiagnosed as having a pinched nerve in their neck or their lower back. In more advanced stages, rigidity may cause an uncomfortable feeling in the muscles of the chest or of the abdominal wall, which sometimes leads to emergency consultations to rule out a heart attack. Some people with Parkinson's with these symptoms go through many tests and consultations with gastroenterologists to look for ulcers or other intestinal conditions. A word of caution is necessary here. Although many unusual sensations and symptoms can be attributed to Parkinson's disease, people with Parkinson's are vulnerable to cardiac (heart) and gastrointestinal (digestive system) conditions just like everyone else, so they should not just blame any new and unusual symptoms on Parkinson's disease without discussing them with their doctor first.

> **Rigidity** is an increase in muscle tone that makes people with Parkinson's disease look stiff.

Rigidity also contributes to a decrease in the size of hand, arm, and leg movements by decreasing flexibility. This is why many people living with the disease appear stiff when walking, turning, or getting up from a lying or sitting position. Because rigidity causes the muscles to be shorter when at rest, it may also lead to a "flexed" attitude of the arms, legs, or entire body. This effect results in a stooped posture or a sideways lean when standing. A pronounced forward stooping is called **camptocormia**, which is Greek for "crooked trunk." The sideways leaning is sometimes called a **Pisa syndrome**.

Rigidity responds favorably, particularly early on, to drugs. However, sometimes patients may continue to have muscle spasms because of rigidity even when all other symptoms are under control. For this reason, special exercises are often recommended for people with Parkinson's. Details on this type of treatment are found in Chapter 8.

Loss of Balance, Freezing, and Falling

People living with Parkinson's disease may experience a loss of balance for a variety of reasons, but this problem usually happens in the moderate to advanced stages of the disease. The classic teaching is that balance is not an issue for people recently diagnosed with Parkinson's disease. But this statement needs to be taken with a grain of salt. It is well known that 20–25 percent of all people over the age of 65 will experience repeated falls. Thus, losing one's balance is not unusual in the age group that is most likely to be living with Parkinson's disease.

Here is a more accurate statement. In the early stages of the disease, patients are not likely to lose their balance because of Parkinson's disease. However, they may be more likely to trip, not be quick enough to catch themselves, and therefore fall. It is important to point out that *frequent* falls early in the course of the disease should be brought to the doctor's attention because they may indicate that Parkinson's disease is not the correct diagnosis. More details on this can be found in Chapter 5.

As the disease progresses, three things may happen that will increase the likelihood of falling: loss of postural correcting reflexes, freezing of gait, and orthostatic hypotension.

> There are many reasons why people with Parkinson's may **lose their balance** and fall. Therefore, it's always important to discuss falling with the doctor.

Postural instability because of loss of postural correcting reflexes isn't well understood. It is not directly connected to the slowness of reaction that many patients experience, because it sometimes happens to people whose bradykinesia is under excellent control with medication. When this symptom occurs, people with Parkinson's tend to lose their balance for no apparent reason. The person may be doing normal things, such as backing up while opening the refrigerator door or in the process of sitting down. Falling backward (a symptom called retropulsion) is a common occurrence in such cases. Doctors will often do a "pull test" to examine the patient's postural correcting reflexes. With the patient standing in front of the doctor, she or he will give a quick, sharp backward tug on the patient's shoulders. If the patient needs to be caught by the doctor to keep from falling, the test is positive. As the disease progresses, falls due to loss of postural correcting reflexes may become so frequent that some people may fall tens of times every day.

An unfortunate characteristic of this symptom is that it rarely disappears with adjustments of anti-Parkinson's drugs or with brain surgery. The doctor may ask for help from a physical therapist who can assess the need and appropriateness of a gait assistive device or may refer the patient to an occupational therapist to educate the patient and caregiver on things as simple as how to safely put on one's pants or as complicated as what kind of adaptive equipment should be obtained (such as rails in hallways or grab bars in bathrooms). Details on adaptive devices are contained in Chapter 8.

Freezing of gait describes what happens when a person's feet "get stuck to the ground" while she or he is walking. This symptom appears in the moderate-to-advanced stages of the disease, and researchers aren't sure what causes it. Freezing of gait may happen as a person first gets up to start walking, but it may also happen in midstride, especially when the person is turning or going through doorways or narrow passages (as at the checkout lane of a grocery store). Interestingly, freezing is less likely to happen on stairs or when there is a striped pattern on the floor. Some walking surfaces, such as uneven ground or carpets, may make the condition more likely to occur. If freezing happens when a person is trying to pivot or jumping up to answer the phone, it can lead to a fall. Although freezing of gait may not respond to anti-Parkinson's medications, it may be overcome with certain tricks. A physical therapist can teach patients such techniques, which are described in more detail in Chapters 8 and 9.

People living with Parkinson's disease sometimes fall as a result of **orthostatic hypotension** (also called **postural hypotension**). This medical term means that on arising, a person's blood pressure drops precipitously (see Chapter 4 for greater detail). Parkinson's disease affects the autonomic nervous system, which is the part of the nervous system that controls functions of our body that are not under voluntary control, such as stomach and intestinal motility, beating of the heart, and production of sweat and saliva. The autonomic nervous system is also in charge of making sure our blood pressure remains stable when we stand up from a reclining or sitting position. We all have experienced a woozy sensation if we get up too fast, especially if we are a little dehydrated or have been kneeling or bending over. This happens because when we stand up, our blood, responding to gravity, tends to pool in our legs; this can cause less blood to travel to the brain. When this happens, the brain shuts down, and we faint. It is the job of the autonomic nervous system to make sure this does not happen by adjusting the tone of the veins in our legs and the force and rate with which our heart pumps blood.

Parkinson's disease often affects how well the autonomic nervous system does its job. In addition, many of the anti-Parkinson's drugs override the autonomic nervous system's responses, creating a perfect storm that can result in fainting or near fainting. In the advanced stages of the disease, this can result in more falls. In Chapter 7, we discuss medications for orthostatic hypotension, and in Chapter 9, we discuss many strategies to minimize the risk of falls and injuries regardless of the cause of falling (which can vary from patient to patient).

Other Motor Symptoms

Weakness

Muscle weakness is not considered a symptom of Parkinson's disease. This may be because when doctors test muscle strength manually in a person with Parkinson's, they cannot generally detect such weakness. But some patients report experiencing weakness. They may be perceiving bradykinesia and rigidity as weakness: the person may not be able to generate muscle power quickly enough when performing certain tasks. But it is possible that in some patients there is an actual decrease in strength; some studies conducted with specialized equipment have demonstrated slight reductions in the muscle strength of people living with Parkinson's disease. In the more advanced stages of the disease, strength can be decreased further because of decreased use of certain muscles. If left unchecked, such weakness can combine with rigidity to cause muscle atrophy (muscle wasting) and eventually contractures (the development of scar tissue inside the muscles). The result can be fixed positions of the extremities and total loss of elasticity and muscle function. For this reason, even in the most advanced stages of the disease, continued exercise remains an important part of treatment. Healthcare professionals such as physical and occupational therapists can assess the patients' abilities and needs and advise on the type and extent of the exercises that are likely to be helpful.

Dystonia

Dystonia happens when muscles contract involuntarily. When dystonia occurs, muscles that are supposed to work opposite each other get activated simultaneously—a phenomenon called *co-contraction*. This leads to cramplike postures and slow, "tense" involuntary movements of the arms, the legs, the trunk, or the face and neck.

Dystonia is a disease in its own right, separate from Parkinson's disease. When dystonia happens as a symptom of Parkinson's disease, it is called secondary or symptomatic dystonia. Parkinson's-related dystonia and dystonic postures not only may be a symptom of the disease, particularly in younger patients, but also may be experienced as a form of motor fluctuation, similar to dyskinesia (these terms are explained in detail further in this chapter). In the former case, dystonia may happen very early in the morning, when people first wake up and before they take their morning medication, or it may happen when the effect of the drugs "wears off." It may also occur as a side effect of anti-Parkinson's medicine, particularly levodopa. When dystonia happens as a motor fluctuation, it may be difficult for the doctor to decide whether more or less medicine is the correct solution. The doctor will ask for a detailed description, and sometimes the patient will be asked to keep a detailed diary of the timing of this symptom, especially in relation to the timing of the medication. The patient may have to come into the clinic and be observed throughout a cycle of the medication over a few hours.

Dystonia can be painful. Early in the disease, it usually responds favorably to anti-Parkinson's drugs, but later it may not. Sometimes when it appears as a motor fluctuation, it may worsen with medication. In such cases, other medications may need to be added to the treatment, including medications used to treat dystonia the disease. Sometimes, injections of botulinum toxin maybe helpful. Dystonia-related pain usually responds to the treatment of the dystonia, but over-the-counter painkillers may also be helpful.

Akinesia

Although **akinesia** is sometimes singled out as a separate symptom, it often is just bradykinesia "gone wild." The word *akinesia* is Greek for "absence of movement." It is used to describe patients who become suddenly unable to move. Patients with akinesia usually experience it in the moderate-to-advanced stages of the disease, and it usually happens in the middle of the night, when a person wakes up and is unable to get out of bed without help. That's one of the reasons doctors may prescribe anti-Parkinson's drug doses to be given at bedtime or sometimes in the middle of the night.

Difficulties with Speech, Voice, and Swallowing

Although most people take speech, voice, and swallowing for granted, they are delicately choreographed motor activities that require fine coordination of many muscles. For most of us, these activities have become automatic from many years of practice. One can almost imagine a computer program somewhere in the brain that gets started and runs speech, voice, and swallowing "on autopilot." However, when the neural hardware that's responsible for tuning all these muscles to the proper pitch or muscle tone ceases to work properly or respond fast enough, these otherwise automatic tasks become a struggle.

That's what happens to many people with Parkinson's disease. Words become slurred and run together (a problem called **dysarthria**); speech sometimes accelerates and loses its expressiveness. Breathing movements are smaller, and the person does not expel enough air to produce a sufficiently loud voice (**dysphonia**). Meaning is not conveyed properly, and as the voice becomes softer and less resonant, it may lose its emotional inflection and content. All these changes, together with loss of facial expression, often make communication very difficult for people with Parkinson's. Problems communicating become a frequent point of friction in couples as each person blames the other's voice or hearing. A person with Parkinson's disease can very effectively correct the problem, especially in the earlier stages, by making a conscious effort to speak loudly and clearly and to separate words. In a way, it's like switching from "auto" to "manual." A speech pathologist may be instrumental in teaching patients useful exercises to encourage this practice; details are discussed in Chapters 8 and 9.

Swallowing is affected in a similar fashion (called **dysphagia**). Most people automatically clear their throat constantly by swallowing saliva as well as all secretions that may be running down the back of the throat from the sinuses and the nasal cavities. This automatic activity slows down considerably in people with Parkinson's disease. As a result, patients may drool and report having thick secretions and feeling like they have a "frog in the throat." Another reason for this annoying sensation is that the many drugs people with Parkinson's may be taking can cause thickening of the saliva. In more advanced stages, the choreography of the swallowing movements may be completely lost, and food may not be easily or properly propelled through the esophagus. As a result, choking can occur when food and liquid slide down "the wrong pipe" and end up in the trachea (commonly called the windpipe). Besides the obvious danger of choking, in the later stages of the disease, dysphagia may lead to aspiration pneumonia (lung infection). When anything other than air goes down the windpipe, one normally starts coughing, forcefully expelling the swallowed item. In the advanced stages of Parkinson's disease, this protective cough reflex may be dampened or completely lost, so that foods and liquids may end up in the lungs without the patient realizing what happened. Such materials may become a breeding ground for bacteria in the lung, which may result in aspiration pneumonia.

There are many treatment strategies to deal with swallowing trouble, as discussed in greater detail in Chapters 8 and 9.

Double Vision

People with Parkinson's disease have many difficulties with their vision, but one frequent symptom is double vision, or **diplopia**. Double vision may happen as a manifestation of various neurologic conditions but can also be part of the natural aging process. When such a problem appears, it should be discussed with and assessed by a physician, because it may not be the result of Parkinson's but may indicate another serious condition. In Parkinson's disease, double vision arises from the inability of the eyes to keep pace with each other, but it may also be caused by dry eyes. Normally, each eye sends the brain a slightly different image because the eyes look at an object from different angles. The brain is capable of fusing the two images into a single, three-dimensional image. When the alignment of the eyes is slightly off, the two images don't merge or they fuse incompletely. In milder cases, this is experienced as a "ghosting" similar to what TV images look like when reception is slightly off. In more severe cases, people see two separate images.

In Parkinson's disease, the muscles that move the eyes do not respond very quickly, and, because one side of the body is more affected than the other, the eyes do not move in sync. This may cause double or blurred vision. In addition, some drugs may impair convergence, which is the ability to bring the eyes close together to focus on an object close to the nose. This "convergence insufficiency" can happen normally as we get older, but some anti-Parkinson's medications may aggravate it. Other anti-Parkinson's medications may reduce the ability of the eye to adjust its focus when looking at objects from afar or close up. People with Parkinson's disease tend to not blink as often as is necessary to lubricate the eyes, and this can lead to a thin film of haze over the eyes. When this happens, vision may be blurry or even double. Surprisingly, sometimes dry eyes lead to excess tear production, so it's possible to have dry eyes and excess tears at the same time, similar to what happens with dry mouth and excess saliva. Dry eyes also become very sensitive to light, and protective glasses may be helpful to reduce discomfort. The use of bifocals, trifocals, or progressive lenses may further compound all these eye problems. Medications are generally not very effective to correct vision trouble, but over-the-counter lubricating eye drops may be helpful with dryness and associated discomfort. A visit to the eye doctor is necessary if simple measures fail.

Other vision problems besides double vision can pester a person with Parkinson's disease. Those are discussed in the sensory symptoms section in Chapter 4.

Apraxia

Apraxia is an inability of the brain to plan and execute certain movements. The term means "inability to act." Medicine recognizes several types of apraxia, and entire books have been dedicated to this phenomenon. Apraxia is not exclusive to Parkinson's disease. It is often seen in people with strokes, traumatic brain injury, and Alzheimer's disease and many other degenerative brain diseases. The person affected may give the impression of having forgotten how to perform certain motor tasks. Some specialists believe that freezing of gait, which affects people in the more advanced stages of Parkinson's, is a form of apraxia. In apraxia, the failure happens at the highest level of command in a person's brain, the part that plans and initiates specific motor tasks. Since this part of the brain is not affected in Parkinson's disease until its later stages, this symptom is usually seen in advanced cases. In fact, the appearance of apraxia early on may be an indication that the diagnosis of Parkinson's disease is not accurate. Although the most common form of apraxia seen in Parkinson's is freezing of gait, other forms may occasionally be encountered, such as apraxia of eye opening, inability to seat oneself, and inability to use utensils.

Unfortunately, apraxia is very difficult to treat. Sometimes physical and occupational therapy may help the patient to develop alternative techniques. Apraxia has become an area of more intense and focused research in recent years, and there is good reason to believe that more effective rehabilitation techniques will be available soon.

Motor Symptoms That May Occur as a Complication of Treatment

Dyskinesia

Dyskinesia is another word derived from Greek. *Dys* means "difficult" or "abnormal," and *kinesis* translates as "movement." Dyskinesia is a word used to describe random-looking involuntary movements. Strictly speaking, dyskinesia is not a symptom of Parkinson's disease. The term is used to describe the involuntary movements that may occur in patients with Parkinson's disease as a "complication" of long-term treatment with dopamine-enhancing medications, especially levodopa. The reason for the quotation marks around "complication" is that the drugs in question cannot be considered the exclusive cause of the dyskinesia. For example, people who receive such medications for reasons other than Parkinson's disease do not develop such movements. Also, it appears that a certain degree of progression of Parkinson's is necessary for dyskinesia to appear. An association exists between the total amount of levodopa a person has received, the duration of such treatment, and the likelihood of dyskinesia. However, it is not clear that this represents a cause-and-effect relationship. It may simply mean that patients with more severe forms of the disease are more prone to develop dyskinesia, but because their disease is more severe, they are also more likely to have received high amounts of levodopa. Another observation is that patients who contract the disease at a younger age are likely to develop dyskinesia earlier; the reasons for this predilection are not understood.

Dyskinesia may take a variety of forms. The most usual form of dyskinesia is **chorea** (a Greek term meaning "dancelike movement"). Chorea may affect the arms, legs, trunk, or even the face muscles (resulting in involuntary grimacing). It may even affect respiratory muscles and result in irregular breathing or gasping. One side of the body may be more affected than the other. When mild, chorea may not be intrusive, and many affected people may not even be aware of the movements. Severe chorea, however, may affect the balance or make it difficult for a person to sit still. Sometimes the movements may even cause a person to fall out of a chair. When the dyskinesia is this severe, it can cause weight loss and serious disability. At times dyskinesia may take the form of dystonia (discussed previously) or myoclonus (discussed in material that follows) and can be painful.

Dyskinesia most often follows the timing of a person's levodopa dosing. Physicians distinguish between two patterns: peak-dose dys-kinesia or diphasic dyskinesia. Peak-dose dyskinesia happens when the blood level of levodopa is at its highest, which is about 30–60 minutes after taking a dose. Diphasic dyskinesia is rarer and occurs as the plasma level rises, so usually within 10–30 minutes after taking a dose; it then disappears as the blood concentration of the drug peaks, only to reappear as the plasma level drops 90 minutes to a few hours after the dose was taken. Often patients have both varieties, and it may be difficult to determine the exact pattern, in which case the doctor may ask the patient to keep a detailed log, recording symptoms every 30 minutes. Some clinics may even bring the patient in for a few hours and observe them through a couple of cycles of medication. Distinguishing between these types of dyskinesia is important, as the appropriate treatment is different for the two types.

As mentioned, dyskinesia is often mild. Even when moderate, the dyskinesia may not cause any functional impairment or pain, and the patient may be only marginally aware of its presence. Since trying to treat the dyskinesia can have a negative impact on other motor symptoms of Parkinson's disease, the doctor and patient may mutually agree not to take any special action. In recent years, physicians have tried to distinguish between "troublesome" and "nontroublesome" dyskinesia before deciding whether an intervention is necessary. Dyskinesia is considered troublesome when it interferes with eating, talking, dressing, sleeping, walking, social interaction, or thinking or when it causes embarrassment.

With peak-dose dyskinesia, the usual treatment involves lowering the amount of levodopa and complementing the lower dose with a different anti-Parkinson's drug. Some anti-Parkinson's drugs may actually improve dyskinesia. With diphasic dyskinesia, the treatment usually involves modifications to the medication regimen that minimize the time that it takes for levodopa levels to rise and fall. More on the management of dyskinesia can be found in Chapters 7 and 9.

Myoclonus

Myoclonus is a type of quick, jerky, involuntary movement that is often seen as a form of dyskinesia in people living with Parkinson's disease. The movements are more sudden than those of chorea. When severe, they may cause people to drop things or even lose their balance. Myoclonus is a relatively rare phenomenon and may respond to special medications, as well as the usual anti-Parkinson's drugs. Sometimes myoclonus happens as a person is falling asleep. This is a normal phenomenon that is called nocturnal myoclonus, but it can be exacerbated by some anti-Parkinson's medications and may be severe enough to interfere with falling asleep.

Fluctuations of Motor Response

Although not strictly a symptom of Parkinson's disease, it's important to address the phenomenon of fluctuations in motor symptoms. Within a few years of starting treatment with levodopa, most people will experience such fluctuations, which may be either predictable or unpredictable. Fluctuations appear in up to 50 percent of patients within 5 years of starting levodopa treatment. The fluctuations are considered a form of treatment complication similar to dyskinesia and may coexist with dyskinesia. The simplest and earliest type of fluctuation to appear is the **wearing off** phenomenon. This means that the symptom relief provided by levodopa fades, or wears off, before the next dose is due to be taken. Usually wearing off is first noticed in the middle of the night after the last dose of the day or early the next morning. It may take the form of decreased mobility or dystonia. Soon, similar wearing off is noticed between doses during the daytime as well.

The reasons for motor fluctuations are not all that well understood, but several mechanisms may be involved. One of the most widely accepted mechanisms is the "loss of presynaptic buffer." This mechanism relates to the fact that any dopaminergic neurons remaining in the patient's substantia nigra have the ability to take up levodopa, convert it to dopamine, and store the dopamine for later use. However, as the disease progresses, more dopamine cells die and the dopamine storage capacity of the substantia nigra declines. Eventually, the only available dopamine is what can be produced immediately from whatever amount of levodopa is present in the bloodstream at any given moment. After a person takes a dose of levodopa by mouth, its concentration in the blood rises quickly, peaking within 30–45 minutes, and then drops to less than half the peak within another 90 minutes or so. As the disease progresses, the drug's effect may last just 1–2 hours. This requires more frequent dosing of levodopa, the use of medications that prolong the presence of levodopa in the blood, or supplemental treatment with other anti-Parkinson's drugs.

As the disease progresses further, other factors may cause unpredictability in levodopa levels (e.g., the rate of its absorption from the intestines or interference with its absorption by foods that are high in protein content). Such factors can lead to unpredictable fluctuations of motor response, which are collectively called the **on/off phenomenon.** In this situation, motor dysfunction, such as dramatic slowing of movement, severe spasms, or tremor, may appear quite quickly and unpredictably in relation to when the medication was taken.

Dyskinesia may coexist with other treatment complications and appear at progressively lower doses of levodopa, eventually leading to what is referred to as the "reversal of the therapeutic window," when side effects such as dyskinesia (which usually reflects too much medicine) coexist with bradykinesia, rigidity, and tremors (which usually reflect too little medicine).

The wearing off and on/off phenomena may also affect a person in other, less obvious ways. When the drug wears off or when the on/off phenomenon occurs, a patient may experience nonmotor symptoms such as generalized pain, chest pain, anxiety, shortness of breath, a panicky feeling, sweating, or severe depression. Such symptoms are considered "nonmotor fluctuations."

CHAPTER 4

The Nonmotor Symptoms

In this chapter, you will learn about

- The nonmotor symptoms of Parkinson's
- The effects of the nonmotor symptoms on body functions
- Nonmotor symptoms caused by Parkinson's versus those related to the medications used to treat the disease

Although the most visible signs of Parkinson's disease are motor symptoms that affect physical activities and functions such as walking, moving, swallowing, and writing, the disease may also cause many nonmotor symptoms that affect the sensory, cognitive, emotional, psychiatric, and sometimes automatic functions of the brain and body. When reading about the nonmotor symptoms discussed in this chapter, it is important to remember that people living with Parkinson's disease will not necessarily experience all of them, and some patients may never experience any.

Sensory Symptoms

Sensory symptoms are those that affect a person's sense of smell, touch, taste, hearing, or vision. Let's start with smell and taste. People with Parkinson's disease often experience a diminished sense of **smell**. Scientific research suggests that the sense of smell may start to diminish many years before a person develops the disease. In an 8-year study of 2267 men, physicians at the US Department of

Veterans Affairs Pacific Islands Health Care Center in Honolulu asked participants to identify the following items using only their sense of smell: pineapple, rose, soap, onion, turpentine, lemon, gasoline, cinnamon, banana, and chocolate. Over the subsequent years, thirty-five of these people (who were an average of 80 years old at the beginning of the study) developed Parkinson's disease. Those who had received lower scores on the smell test were more likely to have contracted the illness.

> Loss of **smell** may be one of the earliest symptoms in Parkinson's disease, sometimes preceding the onset of the disease by many years.

Many people don't realize that most of our sensory responses to food—both positive and negative—are due to our sense of smell. When we arrive home and our partner is cooking dinner, it's the smell of the simmering garlic or onions that gets us excited about the meal we'll soon eat.

> Loss of smell affects our sense of **taste** and causes decreased appreciation of flavor in foods.

Likewise, an unfamiliar smell while eating at an ethnic restaurant we haven't tried before might give us pause. In both instances, our sense of smell leads the way. When we eat food, much of what we taste is interpreted through our sense of smell. The sense of **taste** is limited to sweet, bitter, sour, savory, and salty. So, people who lose their sense of smell also lose some of their sense of taste. When this happens in Parkinson's disease, it may contribute to weight loss. This may be a problem in the more advanced stages of the disease, when the decreased enjoyment of food combines with a slowing in stomach motility (described further in this chapter) to produce a loss of appetite and loss of interest in eating.

Parkinson's disease can affect **vision** in a variety of ways, including loss of contrast sensitivity, double vision, and blurred vision. We discussed some of the vision problems that arise from impaired eye movement in Chapter 3. People with Parkinson's also quite frequently lose contrast sensitivity, which is the ability to distinguish between objects of similar colors based on their different brightnesses. This can lead to problems, for example, if a person is looking for a scuffed-up brown baseball on a brown dirt infield or a red pen lying on top of a red tablecloth. Men and women with poor contrast sensitivity also have trouble seeing objects in dim light.

> **Blurred** or **double vision**, difficulty seeing in **dim light**, and loss of **depth perception** can be frequent problems for people living with Parkinson's disease.

People with Parkinson's disease may have such problems with their vision for many reasons. One possibility is a malfunction of the retina, the inner lining of the eyeball, which is made up of many layers of tissue. The retina contains highly specialized light-sensitive cells and neurons dedicated to communicating the information from these cells to the brain. Based on that information, images are perceived, interpreted, and understood in the brain itself. Scientists have discovered dopamine-producing cells in the retina, so it's possible that some of the visual problems people with Parkinson's experience are related to the dopamine-enhancing medications they take. Some anti-Parkinson's drugs can also cause people to experience blurred vision by decreasing their ability to adjust the size of the iris (the opening of the eye) to allow more or less light in and their ability to adjust the focus of the lens in the eye when looking at things close up or far away. This can produce a result similar to an out-of-focus photo or one that is overexposed or underexposed.

Impaired movement of the eyes also has consequences for vision (as discussed in more detail in Chapter 3 on motor symptoms). People living with Parkinson's disease may have double vision or have trouble "tracking" when they read. Problems with blurred vision can be worse for people with Parkinson's disease who wear bifocals, trifocals, or progressive lenses because one eye may look through the "far" part of the lens while the other eye is looking through the "near" part. Poor eye coordination may also lead to problems perceiving objects in a three-dimensional fashion and affect depth perception.

All this trouble with vision may lead people to misinterpret what they see. Sometimes, for example, they may see shadows in the margins of their field of vision. When such problems occur at the same time as a cognitive or thinking dysfunction or a psychiatric dysfunction, they may contribute to hallucinations. We'll discuss hallucinations and illusions in greater detail further in this chapter.

Parkinson's disease does not, as a rule, affect the sense of **touch**. However, people with Parkinson's disease *may* experience unusual sensations such as feeling crawling or tingling in their legs or feet. These may be the result of muscle spasms or restless legs syndrome, a separate disease that people with Parkinson's seem to have a propensity to get. (We'll discuss restless legs syndrome in more detail in the sleep disorders section of this chapter.)

Parkinson's disease doesn't tend to be a disease marked by physical **pain**, but pain does sometimes happen, mostly as a complication in the more advanced stages but also as a symptom of the disease process itself in the earlier stages. In most cases, pain is caused by stiffening of the muscles. Sometimes this can lead to quite unusual and alarming sensations, such as chest or abdominal pain; one possible cause is stiffness of the chest-wall or abdominal-wall muscles. A patient who experiences such pains may need to visit a cardiologist or gastroenterologist to make sure nothing is wrong with her or his heart, stomach, or intestines. These pains could hide other more serious or even life-threatening diseases (e.g., a heart attack or stomach ulcers). Therefore, they should not be dismissed as an expected symptom of Parkinson's disease without discussion with a qualified healthcare professional.

Rarely, people with Parkinson's may experience otherwise unexplained pain. Some experts have speculated that the neurodegenerative process of Parkinson's disease can spread to a part of the brain responsible for sensing pain, causing what is known as central pain syndrome. This syndrome is similar to what happens sometimes (also rarely) to people who have experienced strokes and is usually treated with medications that have been specifically studied for the syndrome.

Cognitive Symptoms

Another category of nonmotor symptoms of Parkinson's disease is **cognitive** symptoms, or symptoms that have to do with thinking. This category includes effects on attention; concentration; memory; communication using spoken and written language; the ability to make sound judgments, make decisions, solve problems, perform simple math, process new information, and detect and correct one's own mistakes; and self-awareness about one's own physical and mental condition and limitations.

> Mild **cognitive difficulties** can be present even in the earliest stages of Parkinson's disease and should not be confused with dementia.

One cognitive function that is frequently affected in Parkinson's disease—sometimes early in the course of the disease—is the **executive function** of the brain. Executive function includes the ability to make decisions, solve problems, and multitask. A big part of our executive function is working memory, the ability to maintain important information in our brain while we're engaged in complex tasks. For example, a healthy person is usually able to cook and read a recipe at the same time. While reading the next steps in a complex recipe, the cook can remember to stir the vegetables that are gently sautéing in the pan. However, a person with Parkinson's disease may have trouble juggling these two tasks because of a lapse in working memory. As the disease progresses, patients may lose the ability to multitask, to perform activities with multiple steps, and to detect and correct their own mistakes. It might take them longer to think through problems and find solutions. All this sounds like a lot of trouble, but in the early stages of the disease, such **cognitive dysfunction** may not affect day-to-day activities in a major way, as one can compensate by slowing down, which happens anyway as a result of the disease. Patients with mentally demanding jobs may feel the cognitive impact of the disease sooner than others. Doctors use the term **dementia** to describe cognitive dysfunction of sufficient severity to cause major disruption in a person's day-to-day activities to the point that the person cannot continue his or her job and may need help with everyday tasks such as paying bills or managing simple finances (e.g., balancing a checkbook). To count as dementia, the dysfunction has to represent a decline from the individual's previous level of function; be persistent for a certain length of time (usually 6 months); and not be explained by a separate illness, the effect of a drug, or chemical poisoning. Therefore, mild cognitive problems are not necessarily an indication of developing dementia. In fact, doctors sometimes use the term **mild cognitive impairment** to describe cognitive problems that are more than expected for a person's age but not sufficient for a diagnosis of dementia.

A diagnosis of dementia early in the course of Parkinson's disease may in fact lead to a change of diagnosis from Parkinson's to **dementia with Lewy bodies (DLB)**.

A person with dementia often loses short-term memory, has difficulty understanding simple statements and commands, can't communicate thoughts effectively, and loses the ability to perform simple daily activities. About one in three to one in four people with Parkinson's disease develops dementia, but usually not until the later stages of the disease. This type of dementia is called **Parkinson's disease dementia** (PDD). People who experience dementia during the early stages of the disease are often referred to a specialist and may be found to have **DLB**, which is also known as Lewy body dementia or diffuse Lewy body disease. DLB and Parkinson's disease have many similarities but are considered to be separate diseases. The symptoms of PDD are quite different from those seen in dementia of Alzheimer's disease. PDD results from the spreading of the disease process from the brainstem up into the brain hemispheres and out to the cortex, the outer layer of the hemispheres. The cortex is responsible for higher functions of thinking, understanding, putting our thoughts in words, doing calculations, learning, remembering, and using learned information to make sense of a current situation and to act and react appropriately. While Alzheimer's seems to affect the memory and language functions, PDD seems to preferentially affect the executive functions. Eventually, the disease spreads to other areas as well, and, in the very advanced stages, PDD may appear very similar to Alzheimer's. Thankfully, this advanced stage of dementia is seen infrequently in Parkinson's disease.

> **Depression, apathy**, and **anxiety** can be frequent "partners" of Parkinson's disease.

Emotional and Psychiatric Problems

Not all people with Parkinson's experience emotional and psychiatric problems, but it does happen to many people with Parkinson's. The most frequent of these conditions is **depression**, especially around the time of diagnosis. This is not necessarily a reaction to the diagnosis but can be a consequence of the changes that occur in brain chemistry as a result of Parkinson's disease. Depression was found to be a very significant reason for reduced quality of life among people living with Parkinson's disease, second only to the loss of mobility skills. Some researchers theorize that depression in people with Parkinson's is caused by lack of dopamine in the parts of the brain that deal with emotions. It is estimated that nearly one in two people with Parkinson's disease experiences depression.

Depression can dramatically affect a person's quality of life. People with depression feel sad most of the time, may lose their appetite, and may have trouble sleeping, despite feeling tired and sleepy all the time. When severe, depression can be life threatening. Affected individuals may feel hopeless, helpless, or even worthless. All enjoyment and happiness are gone from their life. They may feel that life is not worth living and even attempt to put an end to it. However, qualified healthcare professionals can treat depression successfully, and, in most cases, life-saving help may be just a phone call or an open conversation with a loved one away. It is therefore very important for people with Parkinson's to openly discuss emotional troubles with their doctors.

People with Parkinson's disease sometimes experience a loss of interest without necessarily being depressed, a condition called **apathy**. This problem can be subtle and is sometimes difficult to detect, but it can affect a person's quality of life and interactions with family and friends. Before contracting Parkinson's disease, a person may have been an enthusiastic baseball fan who enjoyed going to games with friends. Although the person is still a fan, now that he or she has Parkinson's disease the person is less likely to call a friend to go to a game. People with apathy lose initiative and motivation; they become less active and more passive. Ask them if they are sad, and they say no. These people still enjoy doing their pre-Parkinson's activities; they just lack the motivation to initiate those activities. As a result, they end up relying on friends, family, and partners to ask them to do things. It's important to understand the difference between apathy and depression. People with apathy may appear sad to their family and friends, but they are not really experiencing emotional distress. On the other hand, people with depression experience serious emotional distress that may lead to loss of appetite, sleep impairment, and a loss of interest in activities.

About half of people with Parkinson's are affected by **anxiety** disorders. Interestingly, some patients had anxiety disorders for years before developing symptoms of Parkinson's. Sometimes the anxiety disorder is related to the wearing off or fluctuations of anti-Parkinson's medication (see Chapter 3 for a discussion of such effects on motor symptoms). In such cases, the anxiety disorder is nonspecific, which means that the feeling of anxiety is not directed toward a specific object or situation but is more of a generalized feeling that something horrible is about to happen. It's almost like going through a "miniwithdrawal" from the medication, and the associated feeling can be quite disconcerting, even frightening at times. When feelings of anxiety result from wearing off, they may be quite severe but are usually short-lived and self-limited.

Parkinson's disease may also be associated with other, more specific forms of anxiety disorders, such as social phobia, an anxiety about interacting with other people, or panic disorder. People with Parkinson's disease may have **agoraphobia**—a condition that causes a person to become nervous or jittery in large, empty spaces or in crowded rooms. Patients can also develop a fear of falling that may confine them to a wheelchair. This may happen after several Parkinson's-related falls: instead of trying to continue walking or learning to walk with an assistive device, the person develops a fear of falling and becomes anxious about walking, despite the fact that he or she still has the physical ability to walk.

Impulsiveness is another psychological condition that some people with Parkinson's experience. It may be triggered by the chemical changes in the brain due to Parkinson's disease, drugs used to treat the disease, preexisting personality traits, or a combination of all these factors. Impulsiveness can lead to excessive gambling, drinking, or shopping or something as simple as leaping up to answer the phone without thinking about one's physical limitations. Impulsiveness can particularly be a problem when coupled with dementia.

Parkinson's disease can also affect a person's **sex life**. People with the disease can experience loss of libido (sexual desire) or an abnormally enhanced libido. This may have to do not only with the disease itself (that is, the loss of dopamine from the brain) but also with the medications patients take to treat the symptoms. Not much is known about the mechanisms through which Parkinson's disease affects a person's sex life and intimacy with a partner. People tend not to be open in talking about sexuality or may be embarrassed by their troubles. However, a 2004 study of seventy-five people found that the majority of women with Parkinson's disease reported difficulties with arousal and reaching orgasm. Many women also had low sexual desire and sexual dissatisfaction. Among men living with Parkinson's, most said they had experienced erectile dysfunction and sexual dissatisfaction. Many men also reported instances of premature ejaculation and difficulties reaching orgasm. Not only the emotional but also the physical aspects of sexuality can be affected by Parkinson's disease. This is discussed further in this chapter in the section on autonomic nervous system dysfunction.

Since healthy sexuality is an important component of life enjoyment, it is important for people with Parkinson's to be open about any such problems with their doctors. Clinicians and researchers who specialize in Parkinson's have been learning a lot about sexuality in Parkinson's disease and will want to know about any sexuality problems because there are many ways to help (see also Chapters 7 and 9).

Another large category of psychiatric dysfunctions in Parkinson's disease is what physicians call **psychosis**, which, in short, means a distorted sense of reality. In people with psychosis, there is a disconnection between one's *perception* of reality and reality itself. This can take the form of **hallucinations**, when a person sees or hears things that aren't there. Less frequently, other senses may also be involved, and then people may feel something touching them or smell or taste things when there is nothing to smell or taste. It can also manifest as **illusions**, when a person misinterprets what he or she sees or hears. Or, psychosis can be more complex, as in paranoia. A person with paranoia may have bizarre or abnormal thoughts and may believe that he or she is being persecuted, is being followed, or is being cheated on by a spouse or partner when in fact nothing like that is actually happening. Such abnormal thoughts and ideas are called **delusions**. Delusions can be very vague and simple or may be very detailed and elaborate.

Hallucinations, illusions, delusions, and paranoia are all symptoms of **psychosis**, a term used to describe a disconnection between a person's perceptions and reality. Dopamine plays a central role in both Parkinson's disease and psychosis.

Psychotic phenomena (i.e., hallucinations, illusions, delusions) may be symptoms of Parkinson's disease or may be caused by medication used to treat its motor symptoms. For decades, researchers have understood that dopamine plays a role in one's perception of reality. Shortly after World War II, **psychiatrists** began treating schizophrenia and other psychotic disorders with medications that fight dopamine in the brain. Many of the people treated in this way developed the physical symptoms of Parkinson's disease, including tremors and loss of mobility. From these experiences, doctors concluded that too much dopamine in the brain can cause hallucinations, illusions, paranoia, and delusions. So, when people living with Parkinson's began developing these kinds of symptoms, doctors believed that the symptoms were side effects of the dopamine-enhancing medications used to treat the disease. However, it soon became clear that some people developed these psychiatric symptoms even on very low doses of the medication. Therefore, it is now understood that the appearance of these kinds of symptoms in people with Parkinson's disease is not only a result of dopamine-enhancing medication but also may be linked to the disease process itself.

One major challenge that physicians and caregivers face is how to help a person with Parkinson's who is exhibiting psychotic symptoms. They are faced with a catch-22 situation: drugs used to combat the psychiatric symptoms lower dopamine levels in the brain, but when that happens, a person may experience more physical symptoms of Parkinson's disease, such as a lack of mobility and increased tremors. Managing this situation requires a careful balancing of medications used to treat motor symptoms with medications used to treat psychiatric symptoms. Because of the central role of dopamine in the mechanisms behind both the motor symptoms of Parkinson's and psychosis, researchers have looked for new directions in treating hallucinations in Parkinson's disease. New medications have been developed that will help a lot of the symptoms of **Parkinson's disease psychosis**, as it is now known, without affecting dopamine actions in the brain. But more on this in Chapter 7.

Sleep

Lots of people have **insomnia**: trouble falling asleep at bedtime or staying asleep throughout the night. Parkinson's disease can complicate a person's sleep in several ways. Many people report difficulty falling asleep. Also, as the disease progresses, the medication used to treat Parkinson's disease may not last long enough. A person may be able to fall asleep but may wake up in the middle of the night or just before dawn because of tremor, muscle stiffness, slowness of movement, or other similar physical symptoms causing discomfort. The person may have a tough time turning in bed or getting in and out of bed. Because the person can't move easily, she or he may have a difficult time getting into a relaxed position to sleep. All these factors can contribute to a poor night's sleep.

> **Sleep disruption, excessive sleepiness,** and **specific sleep disorders** may all be part of Parkinson's disease and may require different treatments. A careful review of any sleep symptoms with your healthcare provider will be necessary to develop the most effective treatment plan.

Another form of sleep disruption people may experience is **restless legs syndrome.** Although this syndrome exists as a separate condition outside the context of Parkinson's, people with Parkinson's disease are very prone to it. People with restless legs syndrome experience a sensation that is difficult to describe, but for many people it feels like an itching, burning, squeezing, pinching, or crawling sensation in the shins and calves. To relieve the sensation, people shake or twitch their legs, or they get out of bed and pace. These unpleasant feelings may happen when a person is sitting in a chair or car, but they seem to happen more frequently when the person is trying to fall asleep. Fortunately, the medications usually prescribed to treat the motor symptoms of Parkinson's disease often help people who are experiencing restless legs syndrome. Some people who have restless legs may have a separate sleep disorder known as periodic movements of sleep. This disorder consists of jerking of the feet and legs while one is sleeping. This behavior may or may not disrupt one's sleep, but it usually affects how well one's partner sleeps.

People with Parkinson's often struggle with **rapid eye movement (REM) sleep behavior disorder (RBD),** a condition that involves hitting, punching, sleep talking, sleepwalking, or some combination of these behaviors as the person acts out dreams (which occur during REM sleep). The problem may be minor and infrequent or disruptive and constant. RBD may appear many years before the onset of

Parkinson's disease. In fact, many specialists consider RBD an early indication that a person may develop a neurodegenerative disease such as Parkinson's. In a 2008 Canadian study of ninety-three people with this problem, twenty-six participants developed a neurodegenerative disease within 5 years. Of those who developed a brain disease, most contracted Parkinson's disease, but several people had DLB or Alzheimer's disease. More recent studies suggested that the proportion of people with RBD developing such degenerative diseases may climb to as much as 70 percent at 10 years for the diagnosis of the sleep disorder.

Sleep may also be interrupted because of **nocturia**, the need to urinate frequently at night. Nocturia may be caused by dysfunction of the autonomic nervous system as a result of Parkinson's disease. It can also be unrelated to Parkinson's. Bladder control difficulties in Parkinson's disease are discussed further in this chapter.

Instead of experiencing lack of sleep at night, some people with Parkinson's disease have **hypersomnia** (excessive sleepiness) during the day. This phenomenon may be the result of the disease or fatigue or may be a side effect of medication. Excessive daytime sleepiness has several aspects besides just feeling sleepy and tired all day. Some people may experience sudden sleep attacks: falling asleep during regular activities without warning. These may be a side effect of dopamine agonists, a class of anti-Parkinson's drugs. (These drugs are discussed in more detail in Chapter 7.) This is why doctors warn patients to avoid dangerous activities, including long drives, climbing ladders, and operating machinery, when beginning new medication.

If a person is sleepy all day, every day, a doctor may recommend that the person be evaluated for **obstructive sleep apnea**, a disorder caused by partial or transient complete blocking of the airway while sleeping. A person with this condition actually stops breathing momentarily—sometimes for as long as 60 seconds—before waking up to take a breath, then resuming sleep. Sometimes, but not always, this may cause loud snoring. These awakenings may happen very frequently (up to hundreds of times in a single night), so that the person never gets deep, restful sleep. Patients may not be aware of how bad the problem is as they do not recall waking up so many times. (To remember that we woke up, we have to be awake for longer than 10 seconds, which doesn't necessarily happen in sleep apnea.) The patient wakes up just long enough to resume breathing and then falls asleep. That's why diagnosing this condition often requires the patient to spend a night in a sleep lab. At the lab, the patient's respiration, brain waves, and blood oxygen level are continuously monitored. Anyone can be affected with sleep apnea, but overweight people are more prone to it. Sleep apnea does not seem to be more frequent in people living with Parkinson's disease than in other people; however, people with Parkinson's may develop sleep apnea even if they are not overweight.

Autonomic Nervous System Dysfunction

The body's autonomic nervous system controls blood pressure, body temperature, heart rate, respiration, movements of the gastrointestinal tract (the stomach and intestines), bladder movements, sweating, saliva production, and other functions that do not require voluntary control. The function of the autonomic nervous system can be impaired both by Parkinson's disease and by side effects of anti-Parkinson's drugs.

Orthostatic Hypotension

Orthostatic hypotension, one of the most frequent problems with autonomic dysfunction, is a dramatic drop in blood pressure when a person stands up. In its milder forms, orthostatic hypotension is experienced as a "head rush" or "dizzy spell." When functioning properly, the autonomic nervous system regulates the tone of smooth muscles inside the walls of the leg veins so that when standing, a person's blood does not pool in the legs. When blood pools in the legs, blood pressure drops, not enough blood makes it to the brain, and the person faints. Because of autonomic nervous system controls, our blood pressure stays the same whether we are lying, sitting, or standing. These mechanisms don't work as quickly in people with Parkinson's disease. In addition, anti-Parkinson's drugs and drugs used to treat some psychiatric symptoms of the disease may also delay or dampen the quick reaction of the autonomic nervous system. In the moderate and advanced stages of the disease, a person with Parkinson's may experience frequent or severe dizzy spells when standing up. He or she may also faint. This is more likely to happen first thing in the morning, when a person rises from bed; after a big meal; or during urination. It's not unusual for elderly men with Parkinson's disease to pass out while urinating in the middle of the night. This is called micturition syncope. One way to avoid this is for the man to urinate in a sitting position.

Because Parkinson's disease affects the autonomic nervous system, it can impinge on many functions of the body not related to the ability to move. It is easy not to realize that **symptoms of autonomic dysfunction** are the result of Parkinson's, so opportunities for appropriate, effective treatment may be missed unless patients bring these symptoms up with their doctors or unless the doctors specifically ask about them.

Gastrointestinal Troubles, Constipation, Nausea, Excessive Salivation, Dry Mouth, and Oral Hygiene

The relationship between the gut and Parkinson's is rapidly becoming a hot topic among researchers looking for the causes and even for a cure for Parkinson's. People living with Parkinson's disease frequently have constipation, both because of the disease and because of the effects of anti-Parkinson's drugs on the autonomic nervous system. **Constipation** happens when the motions of the bowels slow. A similar slowing happens with the movement of the stomach. When food stays in the stomach too long, which is called delayed gastric emptying, it can affect a person's food consumption. Although a person is hungry at the start of the meal, she or he may fill up quickly as a result of this condition. This can lead to loss of appetite, nausea, and weight loss. Physicians treating Parkinson's have observed that people who are diagnosed with the disease often have a history of constipation going back for many years. In fact, in 2009, Mayo Clinic neurologist Rodolfo Savica led a team of researchers who confirmed that people with Parkinson's are 2.5 times more likely than others to have suffered with constipation for as many as 20 years before they were actually diagnosed with the disease. In the early 1990s, **pathologists** started discovering Lewy bodies in the neurons of the autonomic nervous system in the wall of the large intestine of people with Parkinson's. Since the gastrointestinal tract is one of a few ways external agents (chemicals, food, bacteria, or viruses) can gain access inside the human body and given that constipation may well turn out to be one of the earliest manifestations of Parkinson's, a better understanding of the role of the gut in Parkinson's may help identify many possible causes for the disease and could point the way to possible cures. At the time of this publication, our knowledge of this topic is still at the earliest stages, so caution about "new cures" based on the "gut connection" is advised. If people with Parkinson's have questions about any such treatments, they should discuss them first with their Parkinson's specialist.

Anti-Parkinson's drugs can cause **nausea**. These drugs work by adding dopamine to the brain, which helps alleviate the motor symptoms of the disease. However, dopamine may trigger nausea by acting in some areas of the brain that are outside the blood-brain barrier. Many nausea medications work by fighting dopamine. Such nausea medications should only be used very cautiously in people with Parkinson's, and the ones that do not cross into the brain should be tried first.

Excessive **salivation** is a frequent—and sometimes early—symptom of Parkinson's disease. This is a complex problem that results from the combined effects of the disease process on the person's movements as a whole and on the autonomic nervous system's control of saliva production and consistency. Interestingly, studies have shown that people with Parkinson's produce less, but thicker, saliva than those without the disease. However, Parkinson's disease causes a decline in the automatic swallowing of saliva, and the result can be disruptive and embarrassing drooling. Treatments may not always be effective and may cause **dry mouth**, a symptom sometimes worse than the drooling the treatment is meant to correct. There are also some indications that the change in the consistency of saliva may have an impact on the health of the oral cavity in people with Parkinson's. Indeed, oral health is an emerging area of research in Parkinson's disease. We know that the normal bacteria that live in our mouth, which play a very important role in balancing the chemistry of our saliva and aid in digestion and immunity, are different in people who have lived with Parkinson's for many years than those found in the mouths of people without the disease. What this means for not only **oral health** but also the general health of people with Parkinson's is not yet very clear, but every such little deviation from the norm is worth pursuing, as a better understanding may lead in better treatments and better overall health for people living with Parkinson's. For now, it is sufficient to know that it is important to follow meticulous oral hygiene and visit the dentist regularly.

Bladder and Sexual Dysfunction

In addition to the change in bowel movements, bladder emptying may be a problem for people living with Parkinson's disease. Most patients with bladder dysfunction have a condition called **neurogenic bladder**—also known as an overactive bladder—that causes them to go to the bathroom frequently. When combined with slowness in bladder movement, neurogenic bladder can lead to what is called overflow incontinence or urgency combined with incontinence. Several medications can be prescribed to treat this condition, although not always with excellent results. In addition, many elderly people may have other causes of bladder dysfunction, such as an enlarged prostate (in men) or stress incontinence (in women). For these reasons, doctors often may refer patients to a urologist for an evaluation. Failure of the autonomic nervous system can also cause sexual problems, such as erectile dysfunction in men and vaginal dryness and discomfort in women. More research is needed in this area, because medical treatments for bladder dysfunction and sexual dysfunction don't always offer satisfactory results.

Thermoregulation

When a person feels chilly in a warm house or sweats in a cool house, the autonomic nervous system may not be regulating body temperature properly. The process of maintaining the body's temperature is called thermoregulation, and it may be impaired in Parkinson's disease. Hot flushes, sweating episodes, or chills may happen at any stage of the disease but are most often associated with fluctuating response to anti-Parkinson's medications. Abrupt discontinuation of anti-Parkinson's drugs may rarely cause a life-threatening condition resulting from a failure of the thermoregulatory mechanism called the neuroleptic malignant syndrome. In this condition, the muscles become extremely rigid, the body temperature rises abruptly, and muscle fibers may break down, which can result in large amounts of protein "plugging up" the kidneys and causing serious kidney damage. The very high body temperature may also cause permanent brain damage. Although this is a very rare phenomenon, it highlights the importance of discussing any changes in the medication regimen with a qualified healthcare provider.

Fatigue

When a person feels exhausted without having worked, exercised, or run errands, he or she may be experiencing fatigue. This is a separate symptom from sleepiness, although the two may very well be present at the same time. Parkinson's disease causes loss of muscle strength and, in some people, low blood pressure, and these symptoms can contribute to a sense of fatigue throughout the day. Fatigue also can be due to a loss of deep sleep or may be a side effect of anti-Parkinson's drugs. Many other possible reasons exist for fatigue besides the disease itself, such as low plasma levels of certain vitamins or hormonal problems. Increasingly, physicians are recognizing that fatigue can be a symptom of the disease, and often, but not always, a careful interview and examination may lead to the root cause and to appropriate treatment.

Skin Problems

Very early in the history of Parkinson's disease, doctors realized that patients with Parkinson's tended have oily, flaky skin around the eyes, the nose, and the scalp. In fact, one of the earliest scales that doctors used to measure severity of Parkinson's symptoms, the Webster scale, included an item on assessing skin oiliness. This condition is called seborrhea, or seborrheic dermatitis, and is not exclusive to patients with Parkinson's. Treatments vary, but severe cases ought to be referred to a dermatologist.

People with Parkinson's disease may also be at elevated risk for melanoma. Melanoma is an aggressive form of skin cancer that, if untreated, can spread throughout the body and be life threatening. It stems from the melanocytes, specialized cells in our skin and mucosa (the lining of our inner cavities) that contain a pigment called melanin. Melanocytes are responsible for people getting a tan after exposure to sunlight. Since melanin is built from molecules of dopamine, experts have wondered if there is an association between Parkinson's disease, anti-Parkinson's drugs, and the risk of melanoma. A few years ago, a very large and well-designed study demonstrated that people with Parkinson's have an overall higher risk of melanoma than people who do not have the disease. However, in many cases, the melanoma preceded the diagnosis of Parkinson's by many years and was not associated with any use of anti-Parkinson's drugs. Therefore, the scientists who conducted the study concluded that for reasons yet unknown, people with Parkinson's have a higher risk of developing melanoma and that the risk is not influenced by the use of anti-Parkinson's drugs. This observation, however, highlights the importance of people with Parkinson's disease of having regular physicals and even dermatology consultations.

CHAPTER 5

Diagnosis

In this chapter, you will learn about

- The diagnosis of Parkinson's and how it is made and confirmed
- Some medical terminology that doctors use to describe Parkinson's and related conditions
- The role of genetic testing in the diagnosis of Parkinson's
- The role of the various health professionals involved in diagnosing and treating Parkinson's

Barrett was diagnosed with Parkinson's disease at age 31. Arlene was diagnosed at age 46. Both had been experiencing tremors for a couple of years. Barrett's right hand shook occasionally. Arlene's left arm shook most of the time. Although both Barrett and Arlene experienced tremor—a common early symptom of Parkinson's disease—diagnosing them with the disease had to wait until they experienced further motor symptoms.

Making and Verifying the Diagnosis

When assessing a person with Parkinson's-like symptoms, a physician is likely to focus on the person's medical and personal history and to perform an examination, looking for specific clues that will either confirm or disprove the diagnosis. A diagnosis of Parkinson's disease is often made by a primary care physician such as an internist or a family practice physician. Since Parkinson's disease is studied in detail in medical schools, most physicians can recognize the symptoms of the disease fairly readily based on the findings in the examination. However, other diseases may masquerade as Parkinson's disease, so the primary care physician may refer the patient to a neurologist. To make, confirm, or reject the diagnosis, the neurologist will rely on the history that he or she receives from the patient and the patient's family and on the findings of a detailed neurologic examination.

Neurologists apply certain criteria in establishing a diagnosis. Different neurologists may use different sets of criteria. For the most part, the neurologist will want to see at least two of the four cardinal symptoms of the disease that were outlined in Chapter 1: tremor at rest, bradykinesia, rigidity, or balance difficulties, with bradykinesia being one of the two necessary symptoms. Because of the need for consistency, particularly as more and more information has been surfacing about genetic forms of the disease, in 2015, the International Parkinson and Movement Disorder Society published a detailed set of diagnostic criteria for Parkinson's disease that takes into consideration the newest diagnostic methods and genetic information. Although we have more powerful ways to take pictures of the brain to map not only the anatomy but also the function and chemistry of the various brain structures, we still lack a test that will confirm or rule out the disease with 100 percent certainty all the time.

In addition to the typical history and findings for Parkinson's, the examining physician may also look for something called "pertinent negatives." This is medical jargon for symptoms and findings that would not be typical for early Parkinson's disease. On discovering any of these items, the physician may want to reevaluate the diagnosis and proceed with additional tests to look for a different cause for the symptoms. A lot of neurologists refer to these atypical symptoms and findings as "red flags." Such red flags may lead to the diagnosis of **atypical parkinsonism**, or **atypical parkinsonian syndrome**. This is a collective term doctors use to describe a group of brain diseases that share common features and may look very similar to Parkinson's disease.

One such unusual symptom would be extreme balance difficulties with multiple falls during the early stages of the disease. Excessive falling in the early stages may lead to a diagnosis of **progressive supranuclear palsy** (**PSP**), one of the atypical parkinsonian syndromes. Of course, the physician needs to use good clinical judgment because approximately 25 percent of all people over the age of 65 may experience repeated falls. If the falls are unexplained, clearly beyond what one would normally expect for the affected person's age, and happen early in the course of the disease, then the correct diagnosis maybe one of the atypical parkinsonian syndromes rather than Parkinson's.

Another red flag is severe autonomic dysfunction in the early stages of the disease. Severe autonomic dysfunction is evident when a person shows severe and unexplained drops in blood pressure on rising (which may lead to fainting), loses the ability to sweat in hot weather, or cannot control bladder and bowel functions (incontinence). Although such symptoms can be seen in advanced stages of Parkinson's disease, they are unusual in the early stages and, if present too soon, may indicate a different diagnosis, such as **multiple system atrophy**.

Dementia or hallucinations are not usually present when Parkinson's disease is first diagnosed. If these symptoms occur in the early stages, particularly before medications have been started, a physician may consider another diagnosis, such as dementia with Lewy bodies.

In Parkinson's disease, it is unusual for symptoms (e.g., tremor) to affect both sides of the body in a very similar fashion or for the symptoms to affect the midline (like the trunk or the neck) more than the extremities (like the forearm or the foot muscles). One side is usually more affected by the disease, especially early in the disease process. If both sides are equally affected, the physician again may diagnose an atypical parkinsonian syndrome.

Similarly, severe freezing of gait early in the course of the disease— especially if combined with memory loss and complete loss of control of the bowel or the bladder—may indicate an accumulation of fluid in the brain, a condition known as **normal-pressure hydrocephalus**.

The doctor will also have to carefully review medications that the patient is taking because some medications may cause symptoms of Parkinson's without actually causing the disease. These medications include certain major tranquilizers and some medications prescribed for nausea or stomach upset.

Information from the history or findings from the examination may not disprove the diagnosis of Parkinson's disease but may raise questions about whether any other issues must be resolved. For example, while examining a patient for Parkinson's disease, a neurologist may find evidence of other unrelated abnormalities, such as evidence of an old stroke that the patient wasn't aware of. Such a discovery may lead to additional testing, including brain magnetic resonance imaging (MRI) or blood tests. In people with Parkinson's disease, routine brain MRIs appear normal and therefore may not be indicated if the diagnosis is made beyond any doubt. Using specialized equipment and modified computer analysis of the images, brain MRI abnormalities have been found in people with Parkinson's disease. The diagnostic value of such findings is being investigated in ongoing research trials, and it remains to be seen if they will prove of sufficient accuracy for general practice, yet they may help tilt the scale toward or away from a Parkinson's diagnosis.

A lot of information is available on the Internet regarding another advanced diagnostic test based on an imaging technique called **positron emission tomography (PET)**. A PET scan can identify loss of dopamine function in the brainstem in people with Parkinson's disease. If a suspected case of Parkinson's disease shows no loss of dopamine, Parkinson's disease can be reliably excluded as the cause of the symptoms. On the other hand, if the PET scan shows dopamine loss, that doesn't necessarily mean a person has Parkinson's disease. She or he may have any number of atypical parkinsonian syndromes. Therefore, a negative result is significant, but a positive result may not help a diagnosis any more than the specialist's assessment already does.

Another type of a brain scan, called a **dopamine transporter (DaT) scan,** has been approved for diagnostic use in Parkinson's disease. A DaT scan uses a radioactive tracer that "tags" dopamine neurons in the brain; therefore, a "positive" result suggests that the person suffers from a brain disease that attacks dopamine neurons. However, some medications may block the tracer from attaching to the dopamine neurons, creating the false impression of dopamine neuron loss when there isn't any; we call this result a "false positive," meaning the test is positive in the absence of disease.

Since the DaT scan has been around for more than 15 years, Parkinson's specialists have become more aware of people who look like they have early Parkinson's but have a negative DaT scan. Some of these people have shown no progression of their symptoms over the years, confirming that their underlying condition was not the progressive disease we recognize as Parkinson's disease. In these cases, the test was correct, and the doctor was wrong. The reverse has also been seen, especially in the earliest stages of the disease: the test showed no abnormality, yet the person developed the typical disease progression seen in Parkinson's, meaning the doctor was right and the test was wrong.

All this can be very confusing, of course, and it just confirms that the diagnosis of Parkinson's remains a puzzle with many pieces, and that accurate diagnosis sometimes requires a careful review of all the available information by a **movement disorders specialist.** Because of all the intricacies of the diagnostic process (described only briefly previously in this chapter), it is estimated that even with a careful history and examination of the patient, the accuracy of the diagnosis of Parkinson's disease in the early stages is approximately 80–85 percent. That still leaves a 15–20 percent possibility that further progression of a patient's symptoms will show that he or she has a disease other than Parkinson's.

The Role of the Neurologist and the Medical Team

All physicians are fully qualified to make the diagnosis of Parkinson's disease. However, a primary care physician may have doubts and refer the patient to a neurologist for verification of the diagnosis. If there are further questions, the patient may be assessed by a neurologist who specializes in Parkinson's disease. A neurologist of this sort is called a movement disorders specialist. The neurologist and the movement disorders specialist will perform a detailed neurologic examination; they will examine the person's muscle tone, movements, muscle strength, reflexes, coordination, balance, and sensory system function. These doctors may also examine the person's blood pressure in reclining or sitting position and in standing position, and they may perform a brief cognitive evaluation (examination of memory and thinking).

Management of the symptoms early in the course of the disease is generally straightforward whether the patient is on medication or not. During the early stages of Parkinson's disease, patients may decide to see their primary care physician more frequently than their neurologist. As Parkinson's progresses, disease management becomes more complicated, and more frequent visits to the neurologist may be required. In the moderate-to-advanced stages, very frequent visits may be required to readjust the treatment regimen and to manage the increasing complexity of the multiple symptoms that emerge in time.

In the first few visits, the doctor (either the neurologist or the primary care physician) will spend time with the patient trying to explain the disease, the rationale for each treatment, and the prognosis; healthy life choices and the significance of exercise will be reviewed. A physical therapist may review the patient's exercise regimen and may make very specific recommendations. An occupational therapist may provide tips and ideas about how to deal with issues related to daily activities, such as how to get up from a low chair, how to get in and out of a car, how to improve mobility in bed, and how to improve one's handwriting. A speech therapist may become involved if the patient has experienced dysphonia (weakening of the voice), dysarthria (slurred speech), or dysphagia (difficulty swallowing or choking). A speech therapist may also help a patient better understand a drooling problem and how to manage it. If a patient has a partner or close relative, it is generally recommended that this person also be involved in learning about the disease so he or she can provide support and help to the newly diagnosed, now and in the future.

Many people with a recent Parkinson's diagnosis wonder whether doctors recommend genetic testing for Parkinson's disease. Several genes are now known to cause Parkinson's disease. Tests are available for some of these genes, but for many, no tests are commercially available. Therefore, patients can obtain only a partial answer as to whether they have an abnormal type of one particular gene. Moreover, a negative test does not exclude the possibility that the person harbors some other yet-unknown gene that causes Parkinson's. We currently know of at least eleven genes that can cause Parkinson's disease, and many more may not cause Parkinson's but increase one's chances to get the disease; many more are suspected to exist. As of this writing, it is not recommended that genetic testing be undertaken for Parkinson's disease except for very particular cases and for research purposes. The neurologist or the movement disorders specialist will help a patient decide whether genetic testing is appropriate and, if so, may refer the person for further genetic counseling. (Chapter 2 discusses the genetics of Parkinson's disease in more detail.)

Ask the Experts: **Should I Have Genetic Testing for Parkinson's?**

Dr. Martha Nance says, "Although research has shown us that genetics can play a role in determining who gets Parkinson's disease, genetic testing for Parkinson's disease is not yet routinely done in the clinical setting. At least twenty-five different Parkinson's-related genes have been identified, which makes testing complicated and expensive—and most people with Parkinson's disease do not have a mutation in any of the known genes.

"Rare examples have been identified in which Parkinson's disease clearly 'runs' in the family and is directly caused by a specific gene mutation. A person with Parkinson's disease whose family history includes multiple people affected with Parkinson's disease over several generations should consider genetic testing.

"Individuals who develop Parkinson's disease at age 30 or younger are frequently found to carry a mutation in one or both copies of a specific gene called parkin. *Analysis of the* parkin *gene by a blood test would clarify why they developed Parkinson's at such a young age. It may also determine whether other relatives (siblings, children) have a higher risk of developing Parkinson's disease. At this time, the treatment of Parkinson's-related symptoms is no different if the person does or does not have a mutation in* parkin *(or any other Parkinson's-related gene).*

"In the past 5 years, research has identified two particularly interesting and important Parkinson's-related genes: LRRK2 (leucine-rich repeat kinase 2) and GBA (glucosylceramidase beta). Certain variants in the DNA sequence in these genes are strongly associated with the development of Parkinson's disease. Different variants have been identified in different individuals, and some variants are more common in certain ethnic groups. For example, the LRRK2 G2019S variant has been identified in around 10– 15 percent of people with Parkinson's disease of Ashkenazi Jewish descent, while a different variant, L1441R, has been seen in people of Basque descent. Variants in LRRK2 are rare in people of East Asian descent and rarer still in those from sub-Saharan Africa.

"Researchers are particularly interested in LRRK2- and GBA- associated Parkinson's disease, as they have developed specific

treatments to counteract the enzyme deficiencies caused by those genetic variants, and it is possible that those treatments would prevent the progression of Parkinson's disease caused by these genetic variants. The answer to this question awaits further clinical research.

"Some direct-to-consumer companies offer 'genetic testing for Parkinson's disease.' To understand the meaning of a gene test result requires careful attention to details, including what gene (or genes) was tested and how the testing was done. Did the test look for just one specific gene variant (for example, just the G2019S variant in the LRRK2 gene), or was the gene sequenced so as to identify all possible variants? And it is important to understand that the absence of a gene mutation does not mean that a person does not have Parkinson disease!

"The interpretation of gene test results can be difficult. Sometimes a patient is found to have a genetic variant that has never been seen before, and neither the laboratory nor the doctor can say for sure whether that gene variant is related to the disease or not. For all these reasons, genetic testing for Parkinson's disease is not done routinely but is recommended for specific patients or in specific situations (for example, onset of Parkinson's disease younger than age 30, in families with multiple affected individuals, or in certain ethnic groups). Prenatal testing or "predictive testing" (testing of healthy individuals who have a relative with Parkinson's disease) is not recommended, except in very unusual circumstances.

"Another factor to consider is the cost of genetic testing. Insurers often do not pay for gene tests. And while some types of gene tests are relatively inexpensive ('targeted mutation analysis' usually costs less than $500), other gene tests (sequence analysis) may cost $2000 or more. What type of gene test a person should have depends on a detailed understanding of the particular gene

and what kinds of mutations in the gene have been found in people with the disease.

"This is an area of very active research, so the answers to these questions and the use of genetic testing in clinics are likely to change over the next few years. Many families with a history of Parkinson's disease have participated in these research studies, which cannot be successful without their support."

Frequently Asked Questions Regarding Diagnosis and Assembling a Team of Experts

Q: How do I go about choosing the right physician to manage my care?

A: Finding a physician is an important first step in your care. Although your symptoms may be first recognized and treated while you are visiting your primary physician, eventually you may need to consult with a neurologist. A movement disorders specialist is a neurologist who has had specialized training in treating Parkinson's disease and related conditions. Your primary physician may be able to recommend such a specialist, or you can seek out physicians who specialize in Parkinson's by searching websites of regional or national professional associations or organizations of people with Parkinson's disease. (Many such organizations are listed in the Appendix.) Attending a local educational conference on Parkinson's disease may also provide insight into which physicians are involved in the local Parkinson's community.

Building a trusting relationship with your doctor will help you to cope with the disease. The doctor you work with should be willing to answer your questions and take time to explain your symptoms and recommended treatments for your care. Make sure you feel comfortable with the physician's recommendations and that you fully understand prescribed medication schedules and potential side effects. Also be sure your physician outlines a process for how any questions or problems will be handled between appointments and that the physician shares appropriate contact information with you.

Q: *Should I see other healthcare professionals in addition to my physician?*

A: In addition to establishing a trusting relationship with a physician who fully knows and understands current trends in treating Parkinson's disease, it's important to learn about the availability of other professionals who can be helpful. Ideally, these individuals will work closely with your physician to form a healthcare team offering integrated care focused on maximizing options for taking care of your mind, body, and spirit.

The members of your healthcare team will vary depending on your specific needs and the availability of various professionals in your community. Some of the team members' services will be covered by insurance, while others may not. Taking time to learn about resources in your area will help you make good decisions about seeking appropriate individuals who can provide assistance and support when needed. Your physician is a good source from which to begin learning about which resources are in the area, or you can seek advice from a local Parkinson's organization or support group. Your team may include any of the following professionals:

- **Nurse, nurse practitioner, or physician's assistant:** A nurse often works closely with your physician and can be an excellent source for education. A nurse can also provide direction when you are seeking other healthcare professionals (e.g., therapists or social workers) to help you with specific needs. The nurse is often the primary contact person at your clinic and can help you solve problems in person and on the phone. You may also work with a nurse practitioner or a physician's assistant on your team. Nurse practitioners and physician's assistants are professionals with additional training that allows them to perform more detailed evaluations than nurses and to write prescriptions for medications.

- **Occupational therapist:** Previously simple tasks of daily living can sometimes become more demanding or frustrating because of Parkinson's symptoms. An occupational therapist is an excellent resource for learning ways to manage difficulties encountered at home or work. These range from techniques to improve handwriting or the use of utensils to modifications to your home or workplace that will improve safety if your balance is affected.

- **Physical therapist:** A physical therapist specializes in evaluating and treating problems associated with mobility. Physical therapy often helps patients to deal with changes in posture, walking, balance, strength, and endurance as well as other movement-related problems.

- **Speech-language pathologist:** Parkinson's disease often affects communication; many people show a decrease in voice volume, produce imprecise speech, or experience changes in memory. Speech pathologists have expertise in evaluation and treatment of all aspects of communication. They also deal with issues relating to swallowing.

- **Social worker:** A social worker often provides resources and support for coping with a Parkinson's diagnosis. He or she may provide input on available services and insurance coverage and even counsel you on how to deal with challenges in your social environment and workplace. Mental health professionals, such as clinical **psychologists** or **psychiatrists**, may also become involved if additional counseling or medical support is needed.

- **Other therapists:** A variety of other therapists may be involved as members of your team. Music therapists, exercise physiologists, recreational therapists, art therapists, **nutritionists** (also called dietitians), chaplains, and other professionals can lend support in areas of mobility, nutrition, stress management, and spiritual care.

- **Complementary medicine:** Some individuals diagnosed with Parkinson's choose to seek treatment options from alternative or complementary medicine in addition to traditional medical care. Treatments such as massage, acupuncture, and naturopathy are only a few of many complementary therapy options.

Q: Is there a benefit to begin working with a team in early stages of the disease?

A: Yes. Interaction with some team members is likely to be beneficial even in early stages of Parkinson's disease. Although your symptoms may be minimal, it is helpful to learn strategies that emphasize wellness and might minimize or even prevent problems in the future. Some of the newest research suggests that exercise affects the brain, helping to slow brain cell degeneration and maximize the efficiency of remaining dopamine in the brain. Newer techniques used by rehabilitation therapists (physical, occupational, and speech therapists) have been designed to capitalize on the implications of these findings by having patients work on producing large, exaggerated movements and louder voices to enhance and maintain maximal motor function. It appears that these techniques are often most effective in early stages of Parkinson's disease, and the hope is that a person with early gains will be able to maintain them for longer. People with Parkinson's are encouraged to begin other wellness strategies focusing on optimizing general health through nutrition, exercise, and stress management as soon as possible for maximal effect. Preparing for the future through advance **healthcare directives** and financial planning often offers peace of mind to people with Parkinson's disease and their families.

Q: How will I work with my team on an ongoing basis?

A: Members of your team should be willing and available to answer your questions and respond to your concerns at all stages of the disease. This does not mean you will meet with every team member frequently or on an ongoing basis. You may see some team members only once or twice, while others will be involved in your care at more regular intervals. It is often helpful to become familiar with team roles early in your diagnosis so that you have a good idea of which professionals may be most helpful in responding to a new concern. Remember that some team members will need to have a referral from your physician for their services to be covered by your medical insurance.

Q: What should I look for when seeking out professionals for my team?

A: Just as when seeking a physician for your Parkinson's care, it is helpful to ask questions regarding a potential team member's interest, experience, and training in working with people with Parkinson's. Team members should be able to clearly outline their care plans along with any associated benefits or risks of treatment. Therapists should follow standardized practice guidelines of their professional organizations or associations and should be willing to provide you with information and answers to your questions or at least to direct you to another professional who will. Any team member should be clear about expected fees and whether her or his work is likely to be covered by medical insurance. It is often helpful to know how team members communicate with one another to ensure comprehensive and integrated care.

Q: What is my role on the team as a person with Parkinson's disease?

A: Your role is the most important on a well-integrated team. It is important that your viewpoint be expressed and heard as plans for your care are developed. Make sure you are clearly defining your expectations and are working with your team by providing clear and accurate information about your symptoms and reactions to treatment. It may be helpful to write down questions or problems you are experiencing for discussion before going to appointments. Ask for clarifications if you do not understand instructions and make every effort to follow through with recommendations for care, notifying the appropriate person if problems or questions arise.

Q: Should my family or friends be part of my team?

A: Although you will undoubtedly come into contact with a number of new individuals and professionals as you form your comprehensive care team, the people who know you best and love you most are also important members of your team. These are the people with whom you spend most of your time and on whom you rely for daily interaction and support. They may be most acutely aware of your needs and concerns and can provide important insight through their observations. You may wish to involve only one trusted care partner (partner, spouse, adult child, or friend) in your interactions with other team members, or you may wish to have more people involved. In any case, it's wise to bring someone with you to appointments. This person can serve as another set of listening ears, take notes, and allow you to fully interact with the team member you are visiting. It is helpful to have these individuals learn about Parkinson's through participation in appointments, classes, or educational conferences.

CHAPTER 6

How Will My Life Change?

In this chapter, you will learn about

- The immediate impact of being diagnosed with Parkinson's
- Ways that people have dealt with the diagnosis of Parkinson's
- Disclosing the diagnosis to friends, family, and employers
- Taking charge of the situation and the way forward

Being diagnosed with a chronic illness is frightening. It's natural to focus on how Parkinson's disease will make life worse. Undoubtedly, life will present a person living with Parkinson's with many challenges every step of the way, and feelings of despair, disappointment, loss, and being overwhelmed may often darken one's perception of life. Nevertheless, while it seems almost impossible to believe that this unwanted life change could have any positive impact, some people have risen to this challenge, gaining insights and experiencing positive life changes. A relationship with one's partner or spouse may be strengthened. People who stop working earlier than planned may discover time for family, hobbies, and other activities. While being realistic about one's own expectations, strengths, and limitations becomes an essential part of continuing to live a balanced and rewarding life following a diagnosis of Parkinson's disease, there are silver linings, and it is never wrong to try to focus on the positives.

Annie was in her early 40s when she started noticing the subtle symptoms that would turn out to be Parkinson's disease. Here is her story:

"Parkinson's sneaks up on you. Slowly. My first symptoms were anxiety and hand tremors. I remember the anxiety about flying in an airplane, forgetting a meeting, being late, not being prepared for my workday, not reading minds. The tremor was a curiosity at first but not really a hindrance. Today I have less tremor and am more challenged by trying to get my hands to obey when typing, writing a note, or preparing food.

"At the time I first noticed symptoms, my kids were 4 and 6. At work and home, I was very efficient. I was an expert at multitasking, organization, and improvisation. My work environment was flexible enough to allow balance of work and family. As Parkinson's nosed its way in, it stealthily picked away at my methods and my efficiency. I amped up my efforts, lowered some expectations, and kept on this way for several years.

"Gradually, I noticed less and less cooperation between my body and my brain. My movement became more deliberate and slower. Restless legs interrupted my sleep. I had aches and pains, a stiff neck and back. My handwriting, a necessary tool for my job, became tiny and unreadable. Whenever possible, I was in pajamas by 7 PM. I had noticed something was not quite right, and I figured it would pass. I consulted with a neurologist early on. A brain MRI [magnetic resonance imaging] came back 'normal,' so the neurologist concluded my issues were not neurologic in origin.

"I didn't want to believe there was anything wrong with me. I thought the anxiety, tremors, slowness, and restless legs would eventually go away. Our lives were full. We didn't have time to add anything else to the mix.

"A few years slipped by. Family, friends, and acquaintances started to notice physical changes in me. I clenched one fist all the time, lost my arm swing, and dragged a leg when I walked. I smiled less; my facial expressions became stiff. My tremor was more constant. Sometimes friends took my car keys and drove me home from social events, thinking I'd had too much to drink.

I was a teetotaler, but it was obvious at a glance that something wasn't right.

"I needed more time, almost double, to do tasks at work and home. I started getting ready for work the night before, showering, washing my hair, laying out clothes. I skipped breakfast and wearing makeup so I could bank some precious minutes and be on time to work. The house got messier and the meals simpler. I hired someone to help with the housework, a little embarrassed that I couldn't stay on top of it."

On receiving a diagnosis of Parkinson's disease, most people ask, "What will the future look like?" and "Will the disease sap the joy from my life?" One thing we do know is that Parkinson's disease is a chronic and progressive illness. Symptoms and rates of progression vary significantly from one person to another, and there is no straightforward way of predicting one's course with the disease. Your doctor and other healthcare providers will not know whether you wish to learn more or will feel more comfortable knowing less about what the future holds. That's why you should openly share your fears and concerns with your physician and other members of your healthcare team.

Most people have a slow progression of symptoms but still will experience greater challenges as time goes on. To that end, it is important to make realistic plans for the future. Dreams that one may have had for retirement, travel, or one's financial circumstances may need to be reexamined and altered accordingly. It is important to do some soul-searching and look for ways to maintain resiliency and hope as you face this new challenge. No one can see into the future, and none of us knows what each new day will bring. Maintaining open and honest communication with your spouse or partner and trusted friends will help you share your fears, dreams, and plans. A counselor or mental health professional may offer support and assistance in coping with the fear of the unknown. Many people may turn to their spirituality to deal with these feelings and may find comfort and support in conversation with a clergy member, chaplain, or other spiritual adviser.

Reacting to the Diagnosis

A new diagnosis of Parkinson's can be simply overwhelming. Each person reacts to the news in his or her own way. Many people are swept away in a sea of emotions, which may include disbelief, anger, sadness, and denial. Some people have compared receiving the diagnosis to landing unexpectedly in an isolated foreign country with no road maps or knowledge of the language or customs of the area. Others have experienced undiagnosed symptoms for some time and feel that finally receiving a diagnosis is, in some way, a relief. All these emotions are normal reactions to the diagnosis of a chronic illness.

So, where does one go after being diagnosed with Parkinson's disease? It is natural to go through a grieving process. Many people turn to family; friends; and church, synagogue, mosque, or other house of worship for support. Sooner rather than later, most people find the strength to go on. Here is more from Annie:

> *"Five years had passed since my initial neurologist visit. My symptoms were progressing, and my siblings and husband were concerned.*
>
> *"I made an appointment at a new clinic, but I had low expectations for any helpful information. I sat in the exam room, waiting. A silver-haired group of doctors, a postdoctoral learning cadre, paraded in one by one to observe my symptoms and ask me a few questions. They each exited with a tight smile and a nod.*
>
> *"After the parade, the 'real doctor' came in and made a diagnosis. 'I am pretty certain you have Parkinson's disease. But I don't take care of patients with Parkinson's, so come back in a month and see Dr. _____, our Parkinson's expert.' I remember getting*

in the elevator and driving home in light snow flurries. Tremor and anxiety accompanied me. Should I be driving? Parkinson's was an old person's disease. I was 'young.' I hoped the doctor was mistaken (denial). A month was a long time to wait for the expert's opinion and a plan. It must not be that serious.

"I went home and did my research. According to a number of reputable online sources, Parkinson's was exactly what I had. I cried myself to sleep that night. The next morning, I put on my poker face and went to work. A month later, I saw Dr. _____, the Parkinson's expert, who confirmed the Parkinson's diagnosis. I am still grateful for the two and a half hours this doctor spent with my husband and me, discussing and answering questions and setting up appointments with occupational therapy, physical therapy, and speech therapy. The therapy professionals encouraged me to enroll in LSVT BIG therapy, 4 hours a day for 4 weeks. I didn't do it. I had to work and take care of the kids. I thought receiving the diagnosis was the same as dealing with it. I accepted the diagnosis superficially, but I didn't make any life adaptations for it. I merged back onto the freeway of my daily life.

"I was in my early 40s, my symptoms indicated early stage Parkinson's, and I would see Dr. _____ in a year. I was taking a small dose of dopamine agonist, and I used the diagnosis as an excuse to spend time on the couch. In retrospect, I should have done the LSVT BIG therapy; I would have learned a lot, and I would have likely met a support group of peers to help with the questions that worried me. I did not know where to turn for advice, and I didn't realize how beneficial a support group, exercise, and sharing the journey could be.

"Today I know that many of us with Parkinson's wait months to years to have our symptoms labeled. There isn't a cure for Parkinson's, and medications and treatments address symptoms but are not preventive and do not stop Parkinson's from progressing. The quest to label our symptoms gives peace of mind and a 'box' to put it in. The box holds years of information

on Parkinson's past and present. Every question answered leads to a new question to ask. When those of us living with Parkinson's open our boxes and share our experiences, the answers start to catch up with the questions. How fast will Parkinson's disease progress? What are my treatment options? How should I take my medicine? How long can I work? How will we be impacted financially? Should I tell my boss? How do I apply for Social Security? How long will I be able to drive? To walk? Will Parkinson's shorten my life? Will I see my children grow up? Will I have to go to a nursing home?

"I continued to give my energy to work and family, and, when I could, I tried to rest. I was still carrying on as if I didn't have a progressive disease (denial), and, truthfully, I was probably still a bit in the anger and depression stages of grief. I was like a child pinching her ears closed and singing la-la-la-la-la to shut out unwanted sounds. I lived as if I could ignore Parkinson's until it went away."

Seeking More Information

Recently diagnosed people will sooner or later realize that they need to learn more about Parkinson's disease. Scientific studies showed that patients who are better educated about the disease respond better to treatments and manage their symptoms more effectively, in both the short term and long term. An abundance of information is available online. Much of it may be of dubious value, but a lot of it is very useful and informative. Learning more about Parkinson's disease from books such as this or from reliable sources of information such as those listed in Appendix can be very helpful. It will help you understand the disease, ask the right questions of doctors, and be an informed participant in strategizing with respect to disease management. Here is Annie describing her experience learning more about Parkinson's:

"Two years after diagnosis, I learned of a Parkinson's education seminar happening near my house. I went by myself and sat at a back table. The keynote presenter was listing the losses a person with Parkinson's must face. I was not ready for that much reality. I left the room to wipe away tears in privacy. Other parts of the day were more uplifting. Most important, I met a few friends that day. The first was a woman with Parkinson's who helped calm my emotions. The second was a Parkinson's disease nurse who guided me to a clinic where I could participate in frequent community and educational opportunities and support groups and meet "people like me." Attending this seminar was a huge step toward accepting Parkinson's in my life, learning how to advocate for myself, and participating in the Parkinson's disease community."

Reviewing information that discusses every possible symptom of Parkinson's disease can be distressing. It is important to know that while the disease can cause a variety of symptoms, each person is unique and experiences it differently. Avoid the tendency to compare yourself to a person you know who has or had Parkinson's disease, even if that person is a parent or close relative. Symptoms, rate of progression, and response to treatment can vary significantly, especially in comparison with someone who was diagnosed many years ago, when current treatments were not available.

Shortly after diagnosis, some patients decide to get a second opinion. Often people are in denial when first diagnosed with Parkinson's disease. A second opinion may be useful in clarifying any uncertainty in the diagnosis and can be reassuring to patients and their loved ones, even if the diagnosing physician has no doubt. As a rule, physicians are happy to provide a referral for a second opinion and do not see a patient's request for a second opinion as an insult or as questioning their abilities. Physicians often deal with human suffering and insecurity, so they are generally very understanding and willing to provide such referrals on request.

Taking Charge

After the shock of the diagnosis, most people will come to terms with the new reality of having to accommodate Parkinson's as part of their life. The realization comes that life after the diagnosis can be enjoyable and healthy and that most symptoms can be treated successfully or at least managed so that they have a minimal impact on one's life. The uncertainty of how the disease will evolve, as it can be so different from one person to the next, will sooner or later lead to a need to plan for the future. The decision that it is time to take charge and take action comes slowly to some people and may be an epiphany for others. Sometimes people with a recent diagnosis of Parkinson's will be inspired by how others have taken charge of their disease and were successful in maintaining a high quality of life or they may develop a fruitful relationship with a healthcare professional who will show them the way forward. The first question that people may ask once they decide that it is time to take charge of their life again and direct their care is, "What can I do to improve my long-term outlook?" It is true that at the time of this book's publication, we do not know of any medications that can alter the course of the disease. Laboratory research, however, has been pointing to several avenues that may eventually lead to the development of such medications. One way of taking charge is to participate in clinical trials that evaluate new possible treatments for Parkinson's. Many of these experimental treatments will eventually be proven ineffective; however, the more people with Parkinson's agree to participate in such trials, the sooner a breakthrough treatment will become reality. Details about research and how to find out more about it are in Chapter 11.

Scientists have been able to confirm that people with Parkinson's who are otherwise healthy seem to have a slower disease progression. Taking good care of one's other health problems such as high blood pressure or heart or lung problems, following a healthy diet, and developing healthy lifestyle habits can pay big dividends in the long run. But there is more: people with Parkinson's who exercised regularly, at least 2.5 hours a week over several years, were found to maintain a better quality of life that those who didn't. What's more, people with Parkinson's who started exercising several years after diagnosis also saw a long-term benefit in their quality of life. Therefore, it is never too late to start exercising, and, of course, the best time is now. Sometimes it is hard to know where and how to start, especially for those who have not been into exercise all their lives. A healthcare professional such as a physical therapist or a personal trainer familiar with Parkinson's can be a great resource. Here is how Annie described her transition to taking action:

> "About 3 years postdiagnosis, my brother decided to make me his exercise project. Despite using my best deterring tactics, he showed up at my house and escorted me to the health club for exercise every night for several weeks. We did cardio workouts on the elliptical trainer, spin classes, yoga, and weightlifting. The first night I lay on the club floor trying to calm muscle spasms in my back. I'm sure I looked pathetic. Gradually, my body remembered what to do. Within 3 weeks of my new exercise regimen, I felt so much better. My brother thinks what he did for me is no big deal, but really, it was (and is) life changing. I have a positive routine that keeps me in exercise gear instead of pajamas, gets me out of the house, fills a need for being social while improving my physical stamina, lifts my mood, and gives me sense of accomplishment.
>
> "I started to plan my next venture. I saw an opportunity to 'pay forward' the benefits of exercise. I started spreading the news about the benefits of exercise and recruiting others living with Parkinson's to exercise with me. I especially wanted to exercise outside, and research was showing that riding a bike was something people with Parkinson's could do well while enjoying

a respite from their symptoms. I ride daily during the summer months. Some friends ride with me on two wheels, and we cover 25 miles in one ride. Some friends feel more at ease pedaling a shorter distance on supercool three-wheel trikes. Others like to ride with a partner on a four-wheel side-by-side tandem. Riding with friends keeps me engaged in riding. The reward: seeing someone ride successfully when the person thought Parkinson's had taken the fun out of exercise. Their smiles are priceless.

"Through the cold, icy winter months when it isn't reasonable to bike outdoors, I enjoy walking the mall with friends. I also go to the health club—this is how I reset my motivation. My family still keeps me accountable, and I join different classes to make sure I am always learning.

"Reaching out to others living with Parkinson's eased the transition out of my work life, gave purpose to my days, and helped me develop important new friendships. The guidance of the multidisciplinary team at the Parkinson's clinic was also invaluable. Combining their expertise and enthusiasm to sharing the impact and importance of exercise for people living with Parkinson's changed the quality-of-life landscape for thousands of people. I found that through serving and encouraging others to live well with Parkinson's, I was less preoccupied with my own situation. I am so fortunate to be surrounded by positive people—new friends, old friends, family, neighbors, and a health/medical team that cares."

Nobody can pretend that living with Parkinson's is easy. As the disease progresses, a person with Parkinson's and their loved ones can see how it starts to affect one's life in more and more subtle and not-so-subtle ways. How is one to cope, and where does one find the strength to continue the pursuit of a good quality of life? Where does one turn when there is an unexpected downturn or new symptoms arise? Different people draw on different strengths within themselves and their loved ones. Spirituality, humor, purpose, and optimism are some of the strengths people draw on to get through the most difficult times. Support systems may include one's family, religious community, friends, or others with Parkinson's through support groups. The disease itself may color the way people with Parkinson's perceive their own predicament. Apathy, depression, and anxiety may be obstacles to the enjoyment of life, and sometimes help from a professional may be necessary.

Frequently Asked Questions About How to Deal with the Diagnosis of Parkinson's Disease

Q: How will my life change?
A: People recently diagnosed with Parkinson's disease may not notice significant changes to their daily routine. Medications frequently help most of the symptoms, and many people do not feel that their functional status has been altered. It is important for optimal health to maintain good levels of activity, obtain adequate rest, manage stress, and practice wellness strategies. Ongoing participation in leisure interests, social events, and activities that stimulate thinking and good mental health are strongly encouraged.

Some people may experience more prominent symptoms at the time of diagnosis. These symptoms should be thoroughly discussed with the physician and other members of the healthcare team as appropriate. Both physical symptoms and changes in mood and coping skills are of importance and may warrant further examination and treatment.

Talking to your doctor openly about such things as challenges in everyday activities and changes in your work abilities will help you plan better for the future and remove a lot of the stress that stems from the uncertainties of a chronic disease. While assessing what you can and cannot or should not do, it is important to focus on the positive, so that you can enrich your life in the positive areas even as you may be experiencing losses in others.

Q: *How do I tell others that I have Parkinson's disease?*

A: It may be difficult to figure out how to tell your family, friends, and coworkers that you have been diagnosed with Parkinson's. There is not one "best" timetable for doing so; it is a matter of personal preference. It is sometimes helpful to first share the diagnosis with your partner or a close friend who can offer immediate emotional support. You may wish to have simple educational brochures or other resources on hand to share with people you tell of your recent diagnosis to help them understand better what you are going through.

Remember that those you tell will also be reacting to the news and will do so in their own way. You will not have control over their responses and may find that some people need time to process the information, much as you may have when you first received the diagnosis.

Q: *What does this mean for my work situation? Should I tell my employer and coworkers?*

A: You are not required by law to immediately disclose your diagnosis to your employer. While some people feel comfortable sharing this information, others may be concerned that their diagnosis will affect their work relationships with their employer or colleagues. Some people find that attempting to hide the diagnosis from others escalates their stress levels and can lead to exacerbation of Parkinson's disease symptoms.

It may be helpful to speak to a social worker or attorney about your rights under the Americans with Disabilities Act, which protects you and provides you with the right to request reasonable accommodations in your work environment. An occupational therapist can visit your worksite and make recommendations for the accommodations that may be most helpful to you.

If you feel that your disclosure has led to a change in your work status or relationships with supervisors or colleagues, contact the company's human resources representative, seek legal representation, or do both.

If you feel that your symptoms or the medication side effects may lead to dangerous situations, however, it is important to discuss those issues with both your doctor and your employer. For example, if you are a long-distance truck driver and your anti-Parkinson's medications make you sleepy, you need to notify your doctor, your employer, and, depending on where you live, possibly your state's department of transportation.

The Next Step

The next step after you receive the diagnosis of Parkinson's will be to start dealing with the disease. You will need to make decisions about questions such as, When should I consider taking medications? What can I do to help myself? What kinds of changes in my lifestyle will be helpful in the long term? How should I plan for the future? A lot of these questions are addressed in Chapters 7 through 10.

CHAPTER 7

Disease Management

General Principles, Medications, and Surgery

In this chapter, you will learn about

- Different approaches to the treatment of Parkinson's
- How to make decisions about which treatment to consider and at what time as the disease changes over time
- Medications used to treat the motor and nonmotor symptoms and complications of Parkinson's
- Surgical treatments available to alleviate Parkinson's symptoms and how to decide if this is the right treatment

What Are Our Weapons in Treating Parkinson's Disease?

Parkinson's disease is a progressive disease that is currently without a cure. **Medications** can treat many symptoms of the disease successfully, but so far there has been little success in finding drugs that will slow the progression of the disease, much less cure it. Treating the symptoms, however, has allowed most patients to live longer lives. Unfortunately, the effectiveness of medications may decrease as the disease progresses, and the necessary dosages of medications may produce unacceptable complications and side effects. Some of these problems can be addressed through a highly specialized type of brain

surgery called **deep brain stimulation** (DBS), which uses a kind of pacemaker that's inserted into the brain (more on this further in this chapter under Brain Surgery for Parkinson's Disease). As a result of the improved medications and surgeries to treat the symptoms of Parkinson's disease, patients live longer, so the disease has more time to progress. In time, these patients face new challenges for which existing medications and surgical treatments are inadequate. Therefore, doctors and scientists are working not only to find a cure for the disease but also to find treatments for the symptoms of the more advanced stages of the disease, so that the longer lives patients with Parkinson's now have will also have better quality.

> **Medications**, **surgery**, **rehabilitation** services, **exercise**, and specialty **consultations** play complementary roles in managing the symptoms of Parkinson's disease at every stage.

The challenges patients face change with every year that passes. Early in the disease, patients may experience a mild hand tremor, slight stiffness, or a lack of coordination. But as the disease progresses, other symptoms develop, such as decreased mobility, loss of balance, impaired ability to think clearly, and emotional problems. No drugs or surgeries are available to help several of these symptoms, so people with Parkinson's must learn other ways of improving their symptoms with the help of rehabilitation specialists. It's also important that people with Parkinson's and their treating physicians anticipate some of these problems and prepare for what may happen in the future. Even at the time of diagnosis, but more so as the disease progresses, more and more healthcare professionals need to provide their expertise to help patients and their families. These specialists may include physical therapists, occupational therapists, and speech pathologists, who can provide rehabilitation services to lessen the symptoms of the disease. Specialty consultants, such as nutritionists/dietitians, mental health professionals, counselors, and social workers, may help with aspects of a patient's everyday life, including emotional issues and proper diet, and may assess the patient's need for assistance and provide the necessary resources. The health professionals involved in any one person's care will form this person's "team" (see also Chapter 5).

Anti-Parkinson's medications are quite effective in treating most of the disease's motor symptoms, especially in the earlier stages. The decision to start medications to treat the symptoms of Parkinson's disease is usually made when the person with Parkinson's and the doctor agree that the symptoms have reached a point of interfering with the person's life. Sometimes this is not as simple as it sounds.

Many people in the early stages of the disease may be wary of starting mediations, possibly worrying about short-term and long-term side effects. Much of the publicly available information about the effects and side effects of Parkinson's medications may be outdated and can create confusion when patients are trying to make such a consequential decision. It is very important to discuss any concerns about starting medications with your neurologist early. Studies have shown that in trying to avoid taking medication, many people sacrifice quite a bit of enjoyment in life, without much to gain in return.

If, after careful review with the neurologist, a decision is made not to start drugs immediately following the diagnosis, nonmedication approaches to treating the symptoms can still be very helpful. Such approaches may include lifestyle changes; exercise; and physical, occupational, and speech therapy (depending on the types of symptoms a person experiences). Finally, it is important to know that many clinical trials that assess new, experimental treatments that may slow down disease progression often enroll participants in the earliest stages of the disease, when they do not yet require treatment for their symptoms. People with a recent Parkinson's diagnosis who are so inclined should ask their neurologists whether they might qualify for one of these studies. More information about clinical trials can be obtained from reliable online sources. (See Chapter 11 for more information.)

What If I Don't Want to Start Medications Right Away?

Scientific studies suggest that in early stages of the disease, some types of **exercise** may be as effective in controlling the symptoms of Parkinson's disease as some of the available medications. In 2008, Dr. Victoria Goodwin of Peninsula Medical School in the United Kingdom reviewed 342 studies on the impact of exercise on Parkinson's disease. Goodwin found that exercise improved physical functioning, quality of life, leg strength, balance, and walking, but the evidence was insufficient to show effects on preventing falls and the management of depression. In 2017, a group of researchers analyzed the data from almost 3500 people with Parkinson's enrolled in the Parkinson's Foundation's registry. Over three annual follow-up visits, they found that participants who exercised at least 2.5 hours per week had slower progression of their symptoms than those who didn't. More important, participants who started exercising midway through the study were able to slow the progression of their symptoms and maintain a better quality of life.

> **Exercise** may alleviate the symptoms of Parkinson's disease, and there is reason to believe that it also improves the long-term outlook for Parkinson's patients.

The effect of exercise may be more robust than the studies that have been done so far indicate. There are many different ways to exercise, so scientists will try to determine which types of exercise give the most benefit to people living with Parkinson's disease. Although exercise can almost certainly improve some of the symptoms, no one is sure whether it also slows down the progression of the disease. Among the new symptoms patients develop with disease progression, balance problems represent a particular challenge. While scientific studies are insufficient to show definitively that proper exercise early in the disease course can help decrease falls and other problems at later stages, many physicians and therapists who treat Parkinson's disease believe this to be the case.

In a 2007 study published in the *Journal of Neuroscience*, Dr. Giselle Petzinger from the University of Southern California reported some very interesting findings. After injecting mice with MPTP—a chemical that causes Parkinson's-like, dopamine-reducing damage in the brain—Petzinger examined the impact of exercise on dopamine usage in their brains. Half the mice in her experiment exercised on high-intensity treadmills, and the other half did not. Results showed that mice that exercised were faster and had better balance than the ones that did not. Petzinger also found that the dopamine chemistry changes caused by MPTP were different in the two groups. Such evidence leads doctors to believe that besides the beneficial effect of regular exercise on Parkinson's symptoms, exercise may also have an impact on the chemical changes inside the brain of people with Parkinson's disease.

As more studies are done on exercise in Parkinson's, we are finding more surprising effects. Exercise improves not only physical but also mental functioning, and there is reason to believe this happens because exercise activates a brain mechanism called **neuroplasticity**. Neuroplasticity is a process through which the brain develops new pathways, that is, new connections between neurons that may repair or bypass the pathways damaged by the disease. It has become clear in the past few years that exercise helps people with Parkinson's not only by making their bodies healthier and stronger but also by making their brains more efficient. The implication is, of course, that exercise needs to be an integral part of the treatment strategy as early as the diagnosis is established to maximize the long-term benefits for people with Parkinson's. At the same time, it's clear that it's never too late to start.

In the remainder of this chapter, we discuss medications, surgeries, and other procedures that are used to treat Parkinson's disease.

Chapters 8 and 10 discuss rehabilitation, lifestyle changes, and exercise in detail. Strategies to deal with specific symptoms are discussed in Chapter 9.

Medications

Once a decision has been made to start medications, a patient and his or her team need to decide which medication is best. Dopaminergic medications directly affect the dopamine chemistry in the brain in one of two ways. One is to supply the brain with levodopa—a molecule the brain can use to make dopamine. The second approach is to supply the brain with synthetic chemicals that can get in the brain and act like dopamine. These medications are called dopamine agonists. We examine both these classes of medications in the next several sections.

Levodopa

Since its introduction in 1968, levodopa (also called L-dopa) has remained the most popular and effective way to treat the symptoms of Parkinson's disease. The book and the movie *Awakenings* are based on Dr. Oliver Sacks's experience with the use of levodopa when it was first introduced. Levodopa often results in dramatic improvement in the motor symptoms of Parkinson's disease. However, for many patients, the effect of levodopa is not so robust. In some patients with Parkinson's, symptoms such as muscle stiffness and slowing improve appreciably, while other symptoms, such as tremor, do not. Nevertheless, in most patients, levodopa will cause at least a noticeable improvement in most motor symptoms of Parkinson's disease. In fact, when such an effect is not seen, doctors may question whether the diagnosis of Parkinson's disease is correct. Levodopa was used alone when it was first introduced, but now it is almost always used in combination with another medication. In the United States, this other medication is carbidopa.

> **Carbidopa** is an additive that reduces the nausea caused by levodopa.

When used alone, levodopa disintegrates quickly in the liver, lungs, and kidneys. This makes it much less effective. That's why in the early years of its use, its dosage had to be very high—high enough to cause severe nausea and vomiting. In the early 1970s, physicians tried to prevent this from happening by looking for a chemical that blocked the enzyme that broke down levodopa. Several such chemicals were found. Two that are in widespread use are carbidopa and benserazide. The combination of carbidopa with levodopa became widely known under the brand name Sinemet, which is based on a combination of the Latin word *sine* ("without") and the Greek word *emesis* ("vomiting"). So basically, Sinemet means "without vomiting." The combination of levodopa with benserazide is not available for use in the United States, but it is used widely in Europe and elsewhere in the world. Benserazide and carbidopa work in a very similar manner, so the information discussed here applies to both.

> The introduction of **levodopa** in the 1960s is considered one of the greatest advances in the treatment of neurologic disease in the twentieth century.

The addition of carbidopa (or benserazide) to levodopa allowed a number of things to happen. The total dosage of levodopa could be dramatically reduced because a lot more of it made it to the brain and was converted to dopamine. Also, preventing the conversion of levodopa to dopamine outside the brain greatly reduced the nausea and vomiting caused by the levodopa when it was used alone. The combined **carbidopa/levodopa** pills come with two numbers that indicate the dosage of each medication included. For example, one formulation of carbidopa/levodopa is 25/100-milligram (mg) tablets. The first number (25) refers to milligrams of carbidopa, and the second number (100) refers to milligrams of levodopa. Other available formulations are 10/100-mg and 25/250-mg tablets. People who experience nausea with the 10/100 or the 25/250 tablets may do better with the 25/100 strength (more milligrams of carbidopa per milligrams of levodopa). Some people experience nausea and vomiting even with the combination of carbidopa and levodopa. To reduce nausea and vomiting, a doctor may prescribe additional carbidopa beyond what's included in the carbidopa/levodopa pills.

When levodopa was first introduced in the late 1960s, it was heralded as a miracle drug. Unfortunately, the honeymoon didn't last long. Doctors now know that most patients start to experience two undesirable side effects the longer they stay on the medication. One side effect is dyskinesia: involuntary movements such as grimacing, flailing of the arms and legs, or dancing movements of the trunk.

> **Dyskinesia** and **wearing off** may happen after a few years of treatment with levodopa.

The second undesirable effect is that although medication remains effective in controlling, to a degree, most of the motor symptoms of the disease, over time the duration of the effect of each dose becomes shorter. At the beginning of treatment, one can take levodopa two or three times a day and not notice any variability in the amount of symptom relief from one dose to the next. As time goes by, the effect of the medication fades (or "wears off") within a few hours of the patient's taking it. (More details about dyskinesia and wearing off can be found in Chapter 3.)

About 50 percent of patients on levodopa begin experiencing these long-term complications within 5 years of treatment. Dyskinesia and wearing off were observed for the first time in the 1970s (within the first decade of the widespread use of levodopa) and led to the suspicion that levodopa might be poisonous to the dopamine nerve cells whose function it was meant to improve. Although this theory gained momentum in the 1980s, many later studies failed to prove that levodopa is toxic. It became clear that these treatment complications weren't a result of levodopa toxicity but rather indicated a change in the way the brain handles dopamine (and levodopa) as the disease progresses. Nevertheless, the notion that delaying the use of levodopa early on will also delay the onset of complications is strong enough that many people with Parkinson's prefer to suffer more severe symptoms early in the disease to avoid or delay the dyskinesia. Unfortunately, the scientific evidence that such sacrifice will pay dividends in the future does not justify such determination, and most specialists now tend to recommend the use of levodopa earlier in the course of the disease.

Levodopa is also associated with a number of "nuisance side effects." As has already been mentioned, some patients experience nausea. This may present quite a challenge to the physician because antinausea medications work by blocking dopamine and therefore can easily aggravate the motor symptoms of Parkinson's disease. One antinausea drug, however, can't get into the brain: domperidone alleviates the nausea of levodopa without crossing the blood-brain barrier. Domperidone is available in Canada and Europe but not the United States because it has not been approved by the US Food and Drug Administration (FDA). Another strategy to reduce the nausea caused by levodopa is to provide additional carbidopa. Carbidopa is available in the United States in a pill by itself (i.e., without levodopa).

Levodopa is absorbed best on an **empty stomach.**

The nausea-generating effect of levodopa can be decreased by taking the medication with solid foods such as crackers or bread. Many people have found it helpful to use ginger; ginger root, ginger pills, and ginger ale seem to reduce the nausea that's caused by levodopa.

However, levodopa is best absorbed on an empty stomach because it is an amino acid just like the amino acids that make up proteins. When we eat something that is rich in protein, such as dairy products or meat, the proteins are broken down into amino acids in the stomach, which are then absorbed in the first part of the small intestine (the **duodenum** and the **jejunum**). However, the capacity of our body to absorb amino acids is limited, so levodopa has to compete with the amino acids that come from the protein in food. For this reason, doctors generally recommend that levodopa be taken on an empty stomach to maximize the amount that gets absorbed into the bloodstream. This interaction may become more important later in the course of the disease, when people start developing the wearing-off phenomenon. In the early stages, it's probably OK to take levodopa with food to minimize nausea; however, most people can tolerate the drug much better after a few weeks or months, and then it is advisable to switch to taking it on an empty stomach.

Other possible side effects of levodopa (and many other anti-Parkinson's medications) include confusion and sometimes even hallucinations or paranoia. These side effects are not very frequent and happen only in the later stages of the disease. Older people are more vulnerable to these side effects. Just like antinausea drugs, most drugs used to treat hallucinations do so by fighting dopamine in the brain. For this reason, once hallucinations appear, a reduction in the total amount of levodopa may be necessary. Most of the time, doctors recommend other treatment modifications that we discuss further in this chapter under Dopamine Agonists and in Chapter 9.

> Both Parkinson's disease and many anti-Parkinson's medications may cause a **drop in blood pressure**, sometimes severe enough to cause fainting.

Levodopa may also cause a drop in blood pressure. The autonomic nervous system regulates blood pressure when we stand up by fighting the effect of gravity on blood so that the blood doesn't pool in the feet and legs. This reflex action is dampened by levodopa, but it also is dampened by Parkinson's disease itself—in both cases resulting in a sudden drop in blood pressure and fainting when a person stands up, a condition called **orthostatic hypotension**. When a patient experiences dizziness and fainting due to this condition, a doctor may recommend increasing salt intake and drinking more liquids to keep blood pressure from dropping too low, provided that the patient's heart and circulatory system are healthy. The doctor may also recommend the use of elastic stockings to prevent blood from pooling in the veins of the legs or may even prescribe medications that keep the blood pressure up by causing water retention. (Some of these medications are discussed further in this chapter under Other Medications Used in Parkinson's Disease.) With a drop in blood pressure caused by anti-Parkinson's medication or Parkinson's itself, patients taking drugs for high blood pressure may need to have the dosage of such antihypertensive medication adjusted because a lower dosage may now be sufficient to control their pressure.

Finally, people with orthostatic hypotension need to be very careful about how they rise, especially when they get up from bed. They should sit at the edge of the bed and wait a moment before standing. It is generally recommended that men urinate in the sitting position because blood pressure drops during urination. (It is not unusual for men in the more advanced stages of Parkinson's disease to faint when they go to the bathroom to urinate in the middle of the night.)

Some precautions should also be taken when starting levodopa. The doctor should carefully review the patient's medical history. Levodopa may increase the pressure in the eye and aggravate a type of glaucoma called narrow-angle glaucoma. Therefore, patients with a history of glaucoma may need to have their eye pressure monitored carefully while on levodopa. Another situation in which levodopa should be used cautiously is in patients with a history of congestive heart failure. The levodopa dosage should be increased slowly, and the patient should be watched carefully for any reemergence of symptoms of heart failure.

Carbidopa/levodopa is initially prescribed in a regimen of three times a day. The dosage may start with just half a pill three times a day and increase progressively until the symptoms are better controlled. The full effect of a dosage adjustment may not materialize until after a few (generally 3–4) days. As the disease progresses, further dosage adjustments may be necessary. One adjustment is to increase the frequency with which the medication is taken throughout the day. The other is to increase or decrease the individual dose depending on the need to balance the control of symptoms against the emergence of side effects such as dyskinesia. The usual pill formulations are available in both brand name and multiple generic products but are generally color coded the same way: yellow for 25/100 mg, blue for 10/100 mg, and bluish-gray for 25/250 mg.

In the 1980s, a new controlled-release form of carbidopa/levodopa was developed. Called Sinemet CR (for "controlled release"), the drug is available in the generic form under the name carbidopa/levodopa CR. In the earlier stages of the disease, patients can benefit from the CR version of the drug since they need to take it only twice a day, which is more convenient than the three-times-a-day dosing of the regular formulation. Although CR formulations of levodopa have an important role in the treatment of the early and moderate stages of Parkinson's disease, they do not seem as predictably effective in the more advanced stages. As the disease progresses and the long-term complications of dyskinesia and wearing off start to appear, the frequency of the CR formulation must be increased. Under such circumstances, the effects of the CR pills may be a little less predictable than those of non-CR pills because of the less predictable absorption of the medication; at times, CR pills may cause more dyskinesia and at other times more wearing off than the non-CR pills.

One area in which the CR formulation has been quite helpful has been in controlling the symptoms of Parkinson's disease overnight. Patients with Parkinson's disease often experience slowness of movement, stiffness, and inability to get comfortable in bed at night as well as inability to fall asleep if they wake up. Some of these symptoms are improved with a bedtime dose of carbidopa/levodopa CR pills. Another useful application of the CR formulation is for patients who experience nausea, headaches, or dizziness from the regular formulations of carbidopa/levodopa. These symptoms usually occur because levodopa reaches a peak in the blood plasma quickly after the medication is ingested, and then the plasma level slowly drops over the next 2–3 hours. It is during the peak that most people experience the nuisance side effects of the medication, including nausea. With CR pills, this peak is lower and develops more slowly; the decline is also less steep. As technology has progressed and our understanding of how our bodies process the medication has improved, new forms of extended-release carbidopa/levodopa have been introduced. One of them (available in the United States under the brand name Rytary) is in the form of capsules that contain carbidopa/levodopa in beads designed to release the medication in successive "waves," so one capsule can provide multiple successive doses of the medication. This provides a more even "flat-top" profile in how the medication level goes up and stays in the bloodstream, thereby minimizing the "peak-and-trough" effect of the older formulations.

Carbidopa/levodopa is also available in an orally disintegrating tablet form (brand name Parcopa). This pill is easier to take than other forms when no water is readily available, such as when one has to take a pill in the middle of the workday, in a plane or a car, or even in the middle of the night.

As the disease progresses and the duration of the effect of carbidopa/levodopa becomes shorter and shorter, it is natural to think that a means should exist for a continuous administration of the medication. This technology is already used for administering insulin in diabetes, and similar technology was developed for carbidopa/levodopa and Parkinson's. An intestinal gel form of carbidopa/levodopa (brand name Duopa in the United States or Duodopa elsewhere) is administered continuously from a pump (usually carried in a holster or a fanny pack) directly into the duodenum (the part of the small intestine where levodopa is normally absorbed) through a tube that is inserted during a small surgical procedure. This tube is similar to the tubes used to feed people with severe swallowing difficulties. The clinical trials of this pump-administered form of carbidopa/levodopa have indicated that the treatment can provide as much as a 30 percent increase in the time that a person feels they are "on" (i.e., the levodopa has the desired therapeutic effect.)

Besides the typical wearing-off phenomenon, in which the effect of the levodopa wears off before it's time for the next dose, some people with Parkinson's will also experience the on/off phenomenon. When that happens, the effect of the medication simply disappears, as if someone turned off the switch. This can happen at any time, and it can, understandably, be inconvenient and uncomfortable. A powder form of carbidopa/levodopa (under the brand name Inbrija) can be administered through an inhaler. The medication is absorbed quickly through the lungs, bypassing the stomach, and takes effect much faster, getting the person with Parkinson's back to his or her activities within a few minutes.

Researchers have also been developing medications that extend the effectiveness of levodopa by making it last longer in the bloodstream. Such medications block or slow down the breakdown of levodopa and dopamine, and a number have been developed and are available for use. One of these medications is called entacapone and is discussed further in this chapter under Levodopa Extenders. The company that manufactures entacapone has also produced a formulation that contains carbidopa/levodopa and entacapone in one pill.

Dopamine Agonists

Since medical experts first realized that levodopa can cause abnormal, involuntary movements in patients with Parkinson's, scientists have attempted to produce synthetic chemicals that would stimulate the dopamine **receptors** in the brain directly, thus bypassing dopamine. In other words, the effort concentrated on creating drugs that act in dopamine's place. These efforts resulted in several drugs that are collectively called **dopamine agonists**. Some of these medications have been successful in treating Parkinson's disease, while others have been approved for other diseases in which dopamine action is needed but not for Parkinson's. The so-called first generation of dopamine agonists includes bromocriptine (brand name Parlodel). Another first-generation dopamine agonist, pergolide (brand name Permax) has been withdrawn from the market. Subsequent efforts have created a second generation of dopamine agonists. These are pramipexole (also known by the brand name Mirapex) and ropinirole (also known by the brand name Requip). All four of these are available in pill form. The latest dopamine agonist, rotigotine (brand name Neupro), was developed in a patch form so that the medication is absorbed through the skin rather than through the stomach. One more dopamine agonist, apomorphine (brand name Apokyn) is available in injection form and is used for the on/off episodes as a quick fix. A sublingual form of the same medication is under development and is considered experimental. Other dopamine agonists that are used in Canada or Europe have not been approved by the FDA, including piribedil, lisuride, and cabergoline. After many years of use, some patients who took it developed problems with their heart valves. As a result, the company that produced pergolide voluntarily withdrew it from the US market in 2007.

This leaves five dopamine agonists that are currently available for use in the United States: bromocriptine, pramipexole, ropinirole, rotigotine, and apomorphine. The first three, all pills, share certain characteristics. They all have relatively long half-lives, which means that they linger in the bloodstream for a longer time than levodopa. This is a helpful property when levodopa wears off. However, none of these medications is as potent as levodopa in controlling the symptoms of Parkinson's disease; therefore, patients with Parkinson's disease will sometimes continue to experience the wearing-off effect of the levodopa despite the addition of a dopamine agonist.

Another use of dopamine agonists is early on, when symptoms are relatively mild and the full potency of levodopa is not considered necessary. Dopamine agonists are used to delay the need for levodopa and the occurrence of dyskinesia and wearing off. As mentioned previously in the discussion of levodopa, the notion that delaying use of levodopa forestalls those complications is not fully accepted by all Parkinson's specialists. As a group, dopamine agonists can cause nausea and vomiting, and it's usually recommended that patients take them with food. These drugs are usually taken three times a day. Lately, two of them—ropinirole and pramipexole—have become available in the United States in a time-release form that can be taken once or twice a day.

Dopamine agonists have a number of side effects in common, but they also have some individual differences. They can all cause nausea because they stimulate dopamine receptors outside the brain as well as inside. Just like levodopa, they can cause a decrease in blood pressure and may be associated with an increased propensity for hallucinations and paranoia. They may cause confusion, excessive daytime sleepiness, and personality and behavioral changes, swelling around the ankles, and water retention. Not everyone who tries these medications experiences these side effects. However, there are two major side effects that patients and their families should be aware of: excessive daytime sleepiness and personality and behavioral changes. Although these side effects are not always encountered, they may have very serious implications when they occur.

Excessive daytime sleepiness can be experienced either as feeling sleepy and tired throughout the day or as sudden episodes of sleep (also called sleep attacks) that happen without warning during the day. Although the latter form of excessive daytime sleepiness is extremely rare, its consequences can be deadly if the sleep attack happens while a person is driving or operating heavy machinery or in similar situations. For this reason, doctors usually ask patients not to drive or operate heavy machinery during the first few days or weeks of treatment with a dopamine agonist until they know how the medication affects them.

> Sudden **sleep attacks** and personality changes with **obsessive, impulsive, and compulsive behaviors** are two potentially very serious side effects of dopamine agonists.

The second side effect with potentially serious consequences is personality and behavioral changes. Some patients who take dopamine agonists develop obsessive, impulsive, or compulsive behaviors. Such behaviors include excessive gambling or shopping, punding (a term that refers to obsessively taking things apart and putting them together; performing repetitive, seemingly purposeless tasks, such as sorting or rearranging various objects; or collecting trivial items), starting multiple projects and never finishing them, and obsessing about sexual matters. A reduction in dose sometimes helps with such side effects, but if that's not sufficient and the side effect is serious, the medication should be discontinued. When some medication is absolutely necessary, a switch to another drug in the same category (i.e., a different dopamine agonist) may sufficiently control the Parkinson's symptoms without the side effects. If this strategy doesn't work, other medications can be used to control the abnormal behaviors (more on these medications further in this chapter under Other Medications Used in Parkinson's Disease). If the behaviors are neither intrusive nor harmful, simple counseling of the patient and the care partner is sometimes sufficient.

Bromocriptine has one additional potentially serious side effect that may appear after long-term use. This is the development of abnormal fibrous tissue in the abdominal cavity or damage to the fingertips or toes. This complication is extremely rare, but patients and care partners need to be aware of it so that the medication can be discontinued if such signs appear.

Pramipexole is largely cleared from the body through the kidneys; therefore, the dosage may need to be reduced in people who have kidney damage or develop kidney damage. Pramipexole itself does not cause kidney damage. In the presence of kidney damage, however, pramipexole may accumulate in the bloodstream, reaching toxic levels and causing severe side effects, including confusion, severe hallucinations, and sleepiness.

Ropinirole warrants a specific warning: This medication is metabolized (broken down) by the liver. Special enzymes produced by liver cells are responsible for breaking down not only ropinirole but also other medications and nutrients. Among the latter substances are estrogens and the antibiotic ciprofloxacin. Both of these interfere with the breakdown of ropinirole by the liver and may lead to increased side effects from the medication. This is a good example of why it is important to pay attention to any warnings and information that pharmacists supply when dispensing medications.

Rotigotine is a patch that needs to be replaced every day. It is important that the old patch is removed when the new one is applied or an overdose may occur. One particular side effect of this medication is a skin reaction where the patch is applied; therefore, the location of the patch needs to change every day. Sometimes the skin reaction may be severe and affect areas of the body where the patch was never applied; in this case, the medication needs to be discontinued.

In addition to Parkinson's disease, dopamine agonists are used for the treatment of restless legs syndrome. Since patients with Parkinson's disease are also prone to develop this syndrome, sometimes an evening or bedtime dose of a dopamine agonist is added to levodopa just to help control restless legs.

As people get older, they also become more sensitive to the cognitive and psychiatric side effects of dopamine agonists, which include confusion, hallucinations, and paranoia. Therefore, quite often in the more advanced stages of the disease and especially once cognitive symptoms have appeared, doctors slowly withdraw dopamine agonists and focus on maximizing the dosage of levodopa to minimize the risk of side effects.

One dopamine agonist is almost in a category of its own. This is apomorphine hydrochloride (simplified to apomorphine here, known under the brand name Apokyn). Unlike the pills discussed previously, this medication does not get absorbed through the stomach but rather is administered through a subcutaneous injection. It is very fast acting, but its effect also dissipates very rapidly. Because of this, apomorphine is not used for the routine management of Parkinson's disease but rather serves as a "rescue therapy" for people with advanced Parkinson's disease who experience a lot of fluctuations. The term *rescue* simply refers to the fact that an injection of apomorphine may restore mobility in a person whose recent dose of levodopa has worn off and who is not due for another dose for an hour or two; apomorphine rescues the person from having to endure the increased symptoms until the next dose of levodopa. Because the effect of the medication is short-lived, the chance of added side effects when the patient takes the next scheduled dose of levodopa is minimized. Apomorphine has the potential for side effects similar to those of the dopamine agonists described previously. Its dosage should be fine-tuned for each patient. Initiation of treatment with apomorphine takes place in the doctor's office because it is a fairly potent medication and can cause nausea, vomiting, and a severe drop in blood pressure. Some patients may need to take an antiemetic (antinausea) medication in combination with apomorphine injections. Apomorphine is available outside the United States in an injectable form that can be administered continuously through a vein with a pump to try to stabilize the control of motor symptoms in people with Parkinson's who experience a lot of motor fluctuations.

Levodopa Extenders

Another strategy for improving dopamine function in the brain is to use medications that slow the breakdown of dopamine or the breakdown of levodopa. These medications act by blocking certain enzymes in either the brain or the liver, lungs, and kidneys. Two such enzymes have been the target of these medications: monoamine oxidase type B (MAO-B) and catechol-O-methyltransferase (COMT). The classes of medications used to block these enzymes are called **MAO-B inhibitors** and **COMT inhibitors**. Three medications are available in each class. The MAO-B inhibitors are selegiline, rasagiline, and safinamide. Available COMT inhibitors are entacapone and tolcapone. A third COMT inhibitor, opicapone, is available in the European Union. These medications allow the brain dopamine to last a little longer and therefore extend the duration of the levodopa effect, sometimes by as much as 20–30 percent.

> Levodopa extenders work by blocking one of two **enzymes** responsible for the breakdown of levodopa and dopamine; these enzymes are **MAO-B** and **COMT**.

MAO-B Inhibitors

What is most interesting about MAO-B inhibitors is that scientific research suggests that they may slow the progression of Parkinson's disease. This possibility was raised when scientists discovered that MAO-B was found to mediate the toxic effect of MPTP in dopamine neurons. So, in the 1980s, Parkinson's researchers in the United States and Canada began a large study, known under the acronym DATATOP, to see if MAO-B inhibitors would slow the progress of the disease. In 1988, scientists reported that patients with Parkinson's disease who received selegiline for about 2 years had a more benign course of the disease and better symptom control than patients who received a placebo. The study also found that patients who received selegiline did not need to start treatment with levodopa as early as patients who received placebo.

However, the DATATOP study's conclusions were somewhat flawed. Researchers at the time had not realized that selegiline improves the symptoms of Parkinson's disease for weeks *after* the medication is discontinued. As a result, the study's designers had not taken this so-called symptomatic effect into account. So, despite initial excitement about the DATATOP results, doctors progressively became less convinced that selegiline did indeed slow the steady march of Parkinson's disease. Moreover, as selegiline was used more extensively, doctors noted that patients who received the medication experienced side effects such as confusion, hallucinations, and difficulty sleeping. Selegiline is absorbed in the stomach and goes through the liver before it reaches the brain. In the liver, a portion of it is converted into amphetamine-like compounds. These amphetamine-like byproducts of selegiline are blamed for the confusion, hallucinations, and insomnia. Older patients are particularly susceptible to these side effects.

To lessen the shortcomings of selegiline, researchers developed an oral form of the medication under the brand name Zelapar. Zelapar is a tablet that dissolves and is absorbed in the mouth. It does not have to go through the liver before reaching the brain. As a result, the dosage can be decreased to as little as 1.25 to 2.5 mg a day, which is about one-eighth to one-fourth the dosage of regular selegiline. By avoiding the breakdown of large quantities of selegiline in the liver, Zelapar achieves two goals: There are fewer toxic breakdown products, and most of the selegiline makes it to the brain without being lost in the liver.

Another MAO-B inhibitor is rasagiline (Azilect). This medication has a function similar to selegiline, but it lacks many of selegiline's toxic byproducts. Like selegiline, rasagiline is eventually broken down in the liver. Because of this, care should be taken when selegiline or rasagiline is given in combination with other medications that are processed in the liver because interactions between the medications may occur.

The third MAO-B inhibitor to become available was safinamide (brand name Xadago). Safinamide is different from selegiline and rasagiline in some ways. The way it inhibits MAO-B is different, but it also acts on dopamine and serotonin reuptake, so, at least theoretically, it allows dopamine to stay in the synapse longer. Therefore, it has an additional mechanism of making the levodopa effect last longer.

It is thought that MAO-B inhibitors may cause a dangerous increase in blood pressure if taken with certain types of antidepressants, over-the-counter medications, and narcotic analgesics. Similar interactions may occur with certain foods or beverages that are rich in the amino acid tyramine, which is found in aged and fermented cheeses, red wine, and cured and preserved meats. This concern about MAO-B inhibitors is based on the chemistry of these drugs and of tyramine and not on actual occurrences of blood pressure spikes. Nevertheless, MAO-B inhibitors come with a long list of over-the-counter drugs and foods to avoid, although in the last few years the list has been considerably shortened by the FDA. This list is usually supplied by the pharmacist when a prescription is filled and should be carefully consulted when a patient is starting a MAO-B inhibitor. Safinamide has an additional warning that it should not be used by people who have certain retinal disorders, as the medication seemed to cause some retina damage in rats and monkeys.

As soon as rasagiline was available, scientists decided to investigate again the potential of MAO-B inhibitors to slow the progression of Parkinson's disease. In the ADAGIO trial, a 2009 study of more than 1000 patients, researchers found that rasagiline may, indeed, have such an effect. Study participants were treated with rasagiline or a placebo. Two doses of rasagiline were tested: 1 mg per day and 2 mg per day. This large study reached certain conclusions that may, at first sight, appear somewhat counterintuitive and contradictory. The investigators concluded that 1 mg a day of rasagiline did provide a

disease-modifying effect, meaning that patients who received 1 mg of rasagiline a day gained some ground over patients who received placebo for the first 6 months of the study and then started rasagiline. The people who started the rasagiline earlier maintained this advantage over the late starters until the end of the study. However, this disease-modifying effect wasn't observed in patients who took 2 mg of rasagiline a day. Scientists aren't sure why this happened; however, it is known that some drugs do work better at lower doses. Further studies will be needed to determine whether rasagiline is indeed capable of slowing down the progression of Parkinson's.

In practical use, selegiline is taken in a dose of 5 mg in the morning and 5 mg in the early afternoon (to avoid nighttime insomnia and nightmares). Zelapar is administered once in the morning; it dissolves and is absorbed in the mouth. Food and drink should not be taken for a few minutes after the intake of Zelapar. The usual starting dosage is 1.25 mg, or one tablet, in the morning. After 6 weeks, this dosage can be increased to 2.5 mg, or two tablets, in the morning. Rasagiline is given in a pill form, and the usual starting dosage is 0.5 mg in the morning, which can be increased to 1 mg in the morning. Safinamide is taken by mouth once daily. The typical starting dose is 50 mg, increased to 100 mg after the first 2 weeks. All these medications can prolong the effectiveness of levodopa by as much as 20 percent. Because they increase the available amount of dopamine in the brain, side effects may include dyskinesia, nausea, vomiting, hallucinations, and confusion. MAO-B inhibitors are often prescribed early in the disease to treat mild symptoms to conserve dopamine agonists and levodopa for a later time.

COMT Inhibitors

The second class of levodopa and dopamine extenders is the COMT inhibitors, which act through the enzyme catechol-O-methyltransferase. This enzyme is found in the liver, kidney, and lungs as well as in the brain. There are two medications in this category: entacapone (brand name Comtan) and tolcapone (brand name Tasmar). There is also a pill that contains carbidopa, levodopa, and entacapone (brand name Stalevo). Initial studies with these medications showed that patients who experience the wearing-off phenomenon had an increase in "on" time of between 20 percent and 60 percent.

As with the MAO-B inhibitors, the fact that COMT inhibitors block the breakdown of levodopa and dopamine can result in several side effects, including low blood pressure, dizziness, light-headedness, nausea, vomiting, confusion, hallucinations, and sleepiness. Dyskinesia can be exaggerated by these medications. Additional side effects are specific to each of the COMT inhibitors. Both entacapone and tolcapone can cause severe diarrhea, which sometimes eases with continued use of the medication. With entacapone, saliva may turn slightly yellow, and urine may turn a dark orange-brown color. This does not happen to everyone who takes entacapone, but if it happens, it is simply the result of the way the person's liver processes the medication and is not an indication of a serious adverse reaction. It is not a reason to discontinue treatment.

Tolcapone has a potentially serious side effect. It can cause severe, irreversible liver damage that can lead to the need for a liver transplant. Although very few cases with this side effect have been reported, patients who go on tolcapone are required to review warnings of this effect and sign an agreement to receive the medication. Blood tests of liver function should be done before the first dose and then again frequently—every 2 weeks—in the early months of the treatment; later, the frequency can decrease to once a month or every 2 months. A difference between entacapone and tolcapone is that entacapone blocks COMT mostly outside the blood-brain barrier, while tolcapone might also block COMT inside the brain. Another difference is that patients take a 200-mg dose of entacapone with every dose of levodopa, whereas tolcapone is administered three times a day at a dose ranging between 100 mg and 200 mg each time.

> Older medications such as **anticholinergics** and **amantadine** may be helpful in special cases; however, they often have many nuisance side effects, particularly among the elderly.

Anticholinergics and Amantadine

In this section, we discuss medications that do not act directly on the dopamine system. Most of these medications are anticholinergic drugs. The reason for this name is that these medications work against **acetylcholine**, a neurotransmitter in the brain.

Neurotransmitters are chemicals produced in the brain that neurons use to communicate with each other. Dopamine is also a neurotransmitter. Dopamine and acetylcholine have somewhat opposing actions on motor function, regulation of muscle tone, and the production of tremors. Early in the history of treatment of Parkinson's disease, doctors thought resetting the balance between dopamine and acetylcholine in the brain might alleviate some of the motor symptoms of Parkinson's. To reset this balance, doctors used medications that suppressed the function of acetylcholine. These medications were somewhat effective and are still used today.

Unfortunately, acetylcholine has a lot of functions besides regulation of muscle tone, so anticholinergic medications often have many unwanted side effects. For example, acetylcholine is very important in memory functions. As a result, people who take medications that fight acetylcholine may occasionally experience confusion. This is especially true for older people. There have been some concerns raised that long-term use of this class of medications may be associated with an increased risk of developing dementia. Acetylcholine is also pivotal in regulating the autonomic nervous system, so people who take anticholinergics may experience blurred vision, constipation, muscle cramps, difficulty with initiating the stream when they urinate, erectile dysfunction, and sleepiness. Younger people experience fewer side effects when taking these medications, so sometimes anticholinergics are used early in the treatment of the disease, especially if delaying the use of a dopamine agonist or levodopa is desirable.

Medications in this category include trihexyphenidyl (brand name Artane) and benztropine (brand name Cogentin). Sometimes patients will be put on these medications early on and may experience a good effect in controlling motor symptoms. As the disease progresses, however, patients may start noticing more cognitive difficulties. At that point, the doctor may discontinue the anticholinergic medication. In fact, anticholinergics are one of the first medications to go once a person starts to have cognitive dysfunction.

Another medication used for treatment of motor symptoms of Parkinson's disease is amantadine (brand name Symmetrel), which is not an anticholinergic. Amantadine was first produced in the 1960s as an antiviral agent used for the treatment of influenza. Amantadine improves some of the symptoms of Parkinson's in some patients. Initially, it was thought to be quite good for tremor, but it was later noticed that the effect on tremor may fade after a few months. Many Parkinson's disease specialists prescribe it for younger patients who don't want to start levodopa early and who don't tolerate other medications well. Amantadine can cause hallucinations and confusion, especially in older people and the cognitively impaired. It is available in both capsule and liquid form and is usually given twice a day, although some patients can tolerate three or even four doses a day. Side effects may include swelling of the ankles and a rash called livedo reticularis, which makes the skin look blotchy. It may cause dizziness and light-headedness, particularly in older patients.

Over the years, it was noted that sometimes patients who were taking amantadine experienced less dyskinesia than people who weren't. This led to scientific studies that found that dyskinesia responds favorably to the use of amantadine. So lately, in addition to using amantadine in the early stages of the disease, doctors have started prescribing it for dyskinesia. Unfortunately, amantadine does not stay in the bloodstream long enough to provide a sustained benefit in treating dyskinesia in some patients. This has led researchers to look for and develop new formulations of amantadine that may have a more consistent effect on reducing dyskinesia. One such form of amantadine is available under the brand name Gocovri and is taken as two capsules together every evening. The effect starts about 6–8 hours later and may last for the better part of the day. Gocovri has been approved by the FDA specifically as a treatment of dyskinesia in Parkinson's disease. Another extended-release form of amantadine has also been approved under the brand name Osmolex. Amantadine has been used in other neurologic diseases to alleviate fatigue, and some small studies have suggested that amantadine may be helpful in the treatment of balance difficulties. However, clinical experience suggests that in patients with Parkinson's disease, such effects are generally very weak.

Other Medications Used in Parkinson's Disease

As is mentioned many times throughout this book, we now understand Parkinson's disease as a condition that can affect many areas of the brain beyond the dopaminergic neurons and can produce many symptoms that have nothing to do with motor function or with the dopamine levels in the brain. It follows that doctors may use medications besides the ones covered in detail in the previous discussion to treat these symptoms. Generally, these medications are "borrowed" from other diseases and even from medical specialties other than neurology. While some of these medications have been approved for use in patients with Parkinson's, many of them are used "off label" to treat the symptoms of Parkinson's disease. That expression means that the FDA has not given approval for use of the medication specifically to treat patients with Parkinson's disease. Therefore, off-label medications should be used with caution and under the close supervision of a physician with experience in treating patients with Parkinson's.

It is beyond the purpose of this book to examine all these medications in detail, especially since many people with Parkinson's will never need to use most of them. It suffices here to say that whenever a new medication is introduced into your treatment regimen, you and your care partner need to understand the reason for its use, what the desired effect is, and what side effects to watch for. We briefly describe here the classes of medications that are often employed for Parkinson's symptoms that do not respond to modification of dopamine chemistry.

Medications for Tremor

Levodopa, dopamine agonists, MAO-B inhibitors, anticholinergics, and amantadine can be very effective in treating the resting tremor that is typical of people with Parkinson's. However, as many as 20 percent of people with Parkinson's may have a resting tremor that does not respond fully to these traditional anti-Parkinson's medications. Additionally, these drugs may not be very effective for tremor that occurs with action (e.g., writing or reaching for a coffee mug) or with holding something (e.g., holding and reading a newspaper). Faced with such a challenge, the physician may decide to try medications used for treating a different movement disorder called essential tremor, which is characterized by action and postural tremors rather than rest tremors. These medications may include beta-blockers (a class of medications used mainly for the treatment of high blood pressure and some heart problems) or certain seizure medications. Propranolol is a representative of the beta-blockers, while primidone and topiramate are among the seizure medications.

Sometimes tremor is only an intermittent, but still bothersome, annoyance (e.g., when it occurs in social situations and is felt to be embarrassing). In that case, doctors may prescribe a mild tranquilizer, which can be used sparingly and only for problematic occasions. These medications usually are benzodiazepines, the same category as the familiar tranquilizer Valium; these should be used with caution and never be mixed with alcohol. Because they can cause or increase sleepiness, one should not drive or operate machinery when using these medications until their effects are known.

Medications for Insomnia, Excessive Daytime Sleepiness, and Other Sleep Disorders

Sometimes, the reason for insomnia in people with Parkinson's is discomfort from stiff muscles or the inability to get comfortable in bed because of bradykinesia. At other times, tremor may keep a person up or may wake him or her up in the middle of the night when the effect of medication taken earlier in the day wears off. Restless legs syndrome is another frequent culprit. All these causes of insomnia may respond to a bedtime or middle-of-the-night dose of levodopa or a dopamine agonist. If insomnia persists despite such treatments, sleep aids may be used. Over-the-counter sleep aids such as diphenhydramine (known under the brand names Benadryl or Unisom) or the natural hormone melatonin can help. If all else fails, the physician may prescribe an antidepressant that has a sedative effect, especially if depression is also a problem. Older antidepressants such as amitriptyline or trazodone can be quite effective in treating both insomnia and depression in Parkinson's disease, but they may also have side effects. They should therefore be used cautiously and started at a very low dose, increasing the dosage depending on effectiveness and tolerability. Traditional sleeping pills can be used as well, but since most of them can lose their effectiveness with continued use or, what's worse, cause dependence (which means inability to sleep without the pill), they should be used sparingly and under close monitoring by the patient's physician.

Nightmares and rapid eye movement (REM) sleep behavior disorder respond exceptionally well to a tranquilizer called clonazepam. This medication is a benzodiazepine and therefore should be used with caution, especially since it may cause confusion in the elderly. Fortunately, low doses of clonazepam are often quite effective and are usually well tolerated.

Excessive daytime sleepiness may be a side effect of the dopamine agonists or even levodopa, and often a change in the drug regimen will fix the problem. If not, doctors may decide to prescribe medications used for narcolepsy, a condition in which people may fall asleep in the middle of the day without warning. The use of such medicines has not been proven to be helpful in people with both Parkinson's and sleepiness because sufficient clinical studies have not been conducted. Again, a decision for such off-label use of these medications should be accompanied by a careful review of the risks involved and the severity and disruptiveness of the symptom.

Dementia Medications

The past decade has seen a proliferation of medications for dementia, developed primarily for the treatment of Alzheimer's disease. Naturally, the same medications have been assessed for their effectiveness in treating Parkinson's disease dementia. One of them, rivastigmine (brand name Exelon), is the only medication approved by the FDA for that purpose. Rivastigmine is available as both a capsule and a patch. Other medications in the same category as rivastigmine include donepezil (brand name Aricept) and galantamine (brand name Razadyne). All these medications exert their action by enhancing the function of the neurotransmitter acetylcholine. Acetylcholine is to Alzheimer's disease what dopamine is to Parkinson's disease. Medications of this class can improve attention, processing speed, executive functions, memory, and language. As discussed previously in this chapter, acetylcholine works against dopamine, so one might think that using medications that enhance acetylcholine in Parkinson's disease might cause more motor problems. Fortunately, this has not been the case in clinical studies, although these drugs may occasionally cause increased tremors or freezing in some patients. In 2010, Dr. Kathryn Chung of the Oregon Health and Science University led a clinical trial that found that donepezil can reduce falling among people with Parkinson's by as much as 50 percent. Some of the side effects seen with this class of medications are muscle cramping, diarrhea, worsening of stomach ulcers, nausea, worsening of irregular heartbeat, and bad breath.

Another dementia medication called memantine (brand name Namenda) works through a mechanism that bypasses acetylcholine. Clinical studies have shown that memantine is well tolerated by patients with Parkinson's disease dementia and may improve attention, processing speed and executive functions. As patients may sometimes be on a combination of memantine and donepezil, the two medications are available as a combination pill under the brand name Namzaric.

Antipsychotics

Antipsychotic drugs are medications used to treat hallucinations, delusions, and paranoia. The main mechanism of action of these medications is to block dopamine, and all but two have been shown to aggravate the motor symptoms of Parkinson's disease. The two that don't are quetiapine and clozapine. Quetiapine (brand name Seroquel) has been well tolerated by people with Parkinson's in clinical studies but has been found to be, at best, mildly effective. It can cause sleepiness and orthostatic hypotension. Clozapine (brand name Clozaril) has been shown to be more effective than quetiapine in controlling hallucinations and paranoia in people with Parkinson's but has the unfortunate risk of a life-threatening side effect: permanent and irreversible damage to the bone marrow, which may require a bone marrow transplant. Although this complication is rare, it is severe enough that it is now required that patients taking the medication have their white blood cell and neutrophil (a particular type of white cell) counts checked once a week while taking this medication. The frequency of testing may decrease to every 2 weeks after 6 months and to every 4 weeks after the first year of treatment.

Because of the role dopamine plays in psychosis as well as in the motor symptoms of Parkinson's, and since most antipsychotic medications will worsen the motor symptoms of Parkinson's disease, there has been an effort to develop antipsychotic medications that do not block dopamine. One of them, pimavanserin (brand name Nuplazid), has been successful in reducing psychosis symptoms in Parkinson's disease. Pimavanserin's effect may not be immediate, and sometimes people with Parkinson's with psychotic symptoms may need to take this medication for a few weeks until they experience its full benefit. As a general warning, evidence shows that elderly patients with dementia treated with such antipsychotics have a higher risk of being diagnosed with diabetes and may also have a decreased life span compared to patients who do not need such treatment.

Medications for Orthostatic Hypotension

When the person with Parkinson's starts having trouble maintaining a high enough blood pressure when getting up, fainting may occur. The first action the doctor will take is to adjust any blood pressure medications the patient may have been taking and recommend strategies to reduce the problem, which are discussed in Chapter 9. If all else fails, however, the doctor may decide to use medications to increase the person's blood pressure. Such medications include fludrocortisone (brand name Florinef), which increases sodium and water retention; midodrine (brand name ProAmatine), which stimulates adrenaline receptors in the veins and arteries; droxidopa (brand name Northera), which is a building block for norepinephrine, a neurotransmitter similar to adrenaline that is involved in blood pressure regulation through the autonomic nervous system; and even salt pills (sodium is well known to increase blood pressure). Another medication that has been found helpful in treating orthostatic hypotension is pyridostigmine (brand name Mestinon), which is used for myasthenia gravis, a condition affecting the nerve endings in the muscles.

Of course, any attempt to increase the blood pressure may result in increased strain on the circulation (by causing fluid overload in the case of fludrocortisone or by causing the blood pressure to be very high in the reclining position in the case of midodrine and droxidopa). Therefore, these medications require close supervision by the patient's physician. Purchasing a blood pressure measuring device for home use may be necessary, so frequent checks can be done at various times of the day and in various positions (e.g., in bed or standing up). Sometimes, the doctor will give a patient parameters for medication usage. For example, the doctor may instruct that the blood pressure be checked in the morning and the medication only administered if it is lower than a set limit or that a different blood pressure–lowering medication be administered if the blood pressure is too high.

Botulinum Toxin Injections

Quite often, changes in anti-Parkinson's medications, such as adjustment of the dose of levodopa or a dopamine agonist or the addition of an anticholinergic agent or amantadine, will ameliorate dystonia. But when all else fails and depending on the muscles affected by the dystonia, the doctor may recommend botulinum toxin injections. Botulinum toxin is a poison produced by the bacteria that cause a severe muscle disease called botulism that can be contracted from poorly canned foods. This toxin poisons the connection between nerves and muscles, effectively paralyzing a person's muscles. When injected in small quantities in individual muscles, botulinum toxin may alleviate the spasms of dystonia for a few months. The doctor, patient, and care partner must engage in a careful examination of the pros and cons before the decision to proceed with injection can be made. It is important to have a good understanding of what are reasonable expectations. If effective, the injections will need to be repeated every few months (usually every 3 or more months) because the effect is transient. The possible risks and complications vary depending on the site of the injection, the person's other medical conditions, and other medications he or she may be taking. In any case, too-frequent injections should be avoided, as immunity to the drug may develop.

Lately, botulinum toxin injections have also been approved by the FDA for the treatment of excessive salivation in Parkinson's disease. In that case, the drug is injected into the salivary glands.

Medications for Nausea

Nausea is a frequent side effect of many anti-Parkinson's medications. Most of the time starting such nausea-causing drugs at a very low dose and progressively increasing the dose ("start low and go slow") minimizes the nausea effect. At other times, however, doctors may prescribe taking different medications with the anti-Parkinson's drug to minimize nausea. One such antinausea drug is carbidopa (it is available by itself, without levodopa, under the brand name Lodosyn), which is also a component of many pills that contain levodopa. An extra amount of carbidopa (usually 25 mg taken together with or a little earlier than each carbidopa/levodopa dose) may be sufficient to treat the nausea caused by carbidopa/levodopa. Domperidone, another nausea medication, is discussed previously in this chapter in the Levodopa section. For most people, nausea stops being a problem with time. Many other nausea medications can worsen the motor symptoms of Parkinson's disease and should therefore be prescribed with caution and only if absolutely necessary. Sometimes, ginger pills (available at health food stores) help with nausea induced by anti-Parkinson's drugs.

Medications for Constipation

Constipation is a frequent problem among people with Parkinson's disease. A large number of over-the-counter remedies are available for constipation, many of them based on naturally occurring laxatives, such as senna leaves or prune juice. Along with a balanced diet, good hydration, and exercise, these natural substances can help with bowel regularity. Over-the-counter stool softeners such as docusate salts can help patients maintain a softer stool consistency, which also helps regularity. It is advisable to use mild stool softeners on a regular basis to avoid more severe constipation or even stool impaction. More aggressive laxatives (e.g., milk of magnesia, glycerin, or enemas) can be habit forming and should only be used if the patient has had no bowel movement for 3–4 days. One laxative that seems to work well for people with Parkinson's disease when taken on a regular basis is polyethylene glycol (brand name Miralax).

If going for many days without a bowel movement is a frequent occurrence despite a regular "bowel program" as described here, the physician should be consulted. As a rule, fiber-containing, bulk-forming laxatives are not encouraged for people living with Parkinson's disease. These remedies work only if the person takes in enough fluids (eight to ten tall glasses a day). Indeed, not drinking enough fluids while taking these laxatives may have the opposite result and worsen the constipation. For more severe constipation that does not respond to these usual measures, prescription medications, such as lubiprostone (brand name Amitiza) or linaclotide (brand name Linzess), have been shown to be effective as well.

Antidepressant and Antianxiety Medications

As mentioned in Chapter 4, people living with Parkinson's disease often must cope with depression and anxiety. Therefore, it is not at all unusual for them to be prescribed antidepressant and anxiolytic (antianxiety) medications. In general terms, antidepressants belong in one of two major categories depending on their chemical structure and mode of action. One category that is very popular with healthcare providers is the selective serotonin reuptake inhibitor (SSRI) medications. Most people are familiar with the first medication of this class that was ever produced, fluoxetine (brand name Prozac). These medications act by modifying the processing in the brain of a chemical called **serotonin**, which shares some chemical characteristics with dopamine but is involved more in the experience of emotions and pain rather than in mobility. The second big category is the tricyclic antidepressants, named for their peculiar molecular structure. One widely used medication from this category is amitriptyline (brand name Elavil). These antidepressants are older than the SSRIs and work through another brain chemical, **norepinephrine**. Several studies have shown that these older antidepressants are very effective in treating depression in Parkinson's disease—at least as effective as their newer counterparts. In addition to these two categories, other antidepressants are also available, but all of them work through modifying serotonin, norepinephrine, or both.

One common property of all antidepressants important to keep in mind is that their action is not immediate, so the full antidepressant effect may not materialize for several weeks. A number of studies have found that during this early part of the treatment, there may be a slight increase in the risk of suicidal thoughts (or even attempts in some patients); therefore, people who start treatment with antidepressants should be closely monitored for any such feelings. All antidepressants have a variety of side effects. Some tend to cause drowsiness, in which case they may double as mild sedatives in people who also have insomnia, while others may give people a slight nervousness, similar to a slight "caffeine buzz." The older antidepressants tend to have more nuisance side effects, such as dry mouth, blurred vision, increased constipation, or increased trouble with urination. In serious cases, they can cause urine retention, a dangerous situation. In older people, especially those who may experience significant cognitive problems, these medications can cause confusion or even hallucinations. A concern exists that because of their mechanism of action, SSRI antidepressants may interact with MAO-B inhibitors (e.g., rasagiline and selegiline) to cause a dangerous rise in blood pressure. Therefore, such combinations should be used with caution.

Most antianxiety drugs have an addictive potential, an important fact to remember. Just like antidepressants, some anxiolytics may have a sedative effect, but regular use of these medications to induce sleep is not recommended because they tend to lose their effectiveness with continuous use; that leads to higher doses and eventual dependence on the drug. The most common use of anxiolytics is on an as-needed basis, with strict limits that are not to be exceeded without a careful discussion with the physician. The most widely known drug in this category is diazepam (brand name Valium), although newer, less-sedating anxiolytics, such as alprazolam or lorazepam, are now used. One medication in this category, clonazepam (brand name Klonopin), has a special use in treating the REM sleep behavior disorder that was mentioned in Chapter 4 and earlier in this chapter. As with most other medications that affect brain chemistry, these drugs can cause confusion, especially in individuals who are elderly or cognitively impaired. They should never be mixed with alcohol.

Drugs are not always the best solution to emotional problems such as depression and anxiety. Because of the different ways insurance companies cover mental health problems, often it is the family physician or the neurologist who decides how to treat such issues. However, it's always best to ask the experts, so if medications are not effective in alleviating these problems, a consultation with a psychiatrist or possibly a psychotherapist should be pursued.

Medications for Excessive Salivation and for Thick Secretions

Drugs that decrease the amount of saliva also make saliva and other secretions thicker. Because this can be quite uncomfortable, using medications to control drooling is reserved for severe cases or special occasions. Some people with Parkinson's disease may use drops or pills that reduce salivation as needed, for example, for social outings, going to church, or visiting with friends. The most frequently used pills are glycopyrrolate (brand name Robinul) and hyoscyamine (brand name Levsin); drops may use atropine. All these medications can cause side effects such as blurred vision, constipation, nausea, erectile dysfunction, decreased sweating, and irregular heartbeat; therefore, they should be used sparingly. Botulinum toxin injections into the salivary glands have also been effective in decreasing saliva production, but on rare occasions, they have the unwanted complication of temporarily worsening swallowing.

Some persons with Parkinson's have the opposite problem from excessive saliva. They develop thick secretions and have trouble clearing their throat or are bothered by thick postnasal drip. Over-the-counter preparations such as guaifenesin (brand name Mucinex), adequate hydration, and a space humidifier may be helpful measures for thick secretions.

Medications to Improve Bladder Control and Erectile Function

People living with Parkinson's disease may experience urgency and frequency of urination and often have to get up a lot at night to go to the bathroom. Although a number of medications are effective in treating these symptoms, these same medications may worsen a person's ability to relax the bladder to start the urinary stream. In a man with prostate trouble, this can cause urinary retention, which is a serious condition. Therefore, it's best to first try to manage the bladder symptoms as much as possible without medications. Some of the nondrug treatments for bladder control are discussed in Chapter 9.

Most medicines used to control this bladder overactivity work by blocking the effect of acetylcholine. If you have read the information presented so far in this chapter, you have learned that drugs that block acetylcholine may have unpleasant side effects, such as confusion, blurred vision, increased constipation, and dry mouth. Medications commonly used for bladder control include oxybutynin (brand name Ditropan), tolterodine (brand name Detrol), and propantheline (brand name Pro-Banthine), but a number of newer medications in the same category are also available. Mirabegron (brand name Myrbetriq), a newer medication for overactive bladder, bypasses acetylcholine and allows the bladder to relax and accommodate more urine before a person has to urinate. In clinical trials, it has been shown to be a safe and effective treatment of overactive bladder symptoms in Parkinson's disease. If starting the urine stream is difficult, doctors may sometimes prescribe tamsulosin (brand name Flomax), which may make urination easier but can often cause a drop in blood pressure. Conversely, some of the medications used to keep blood pressure high may make bladder emptying more difficult. One such medication is midodrine, which was discussed in the section on drugs for orthostatic hypotension.

As mentioned in Chapter 4, people living with Parkinson's disease may experience increased difficulties with their sexual abilities. Many people are reluctant to discuss this problem openly. However, a healthy sex life is an important component of a person's quality of life. Since help may be available, it is important to discuss such problems with your doctor. Medications commonly used to treat erectile dysfunction, such as sildenafil (brand name Viagra), vardenafil (Levitra), and tadalafil (Cialis), can be effective in men with Parkinson's disease. Three things, however, are very important to know before using these medications. First, your doctor will need to review all your other medications. Some medications used in Parkinson's disease (e.g., propranolol, a beta-blocker sometimes used to treat tremor) may cause erectile dysfunction, so the solution may be as simple as skipping a dose of that medication when anticipating intercourse (but you should *not* skip doses of any medications without permission from your doctor). Second, any psychological factors should be discussed and treated: depression is a common cause of decreased sexual desire and erectile dysfunction. And third, you should have a detailed discussion with your doctor about the risks of using these medications, and you should make sure your doctor is aware of any heart trouble you may have before prescribing them.

Some anti-Parkinson's medications, particularly the dopamine agonists pramipexole and ropinirole, may cause increased sexual desire and even obsessing about sex. This can be a serious side effect, as it may create serious difficulties with intimacy in couples affected by Parkinson's. It is important to recognize and discuss such trouble with your doctor. A decrease in dosage may be all that's necessary to deal with this issue, but when the problem is severe, the medication should be discontinued completely. If that's not possible without a serious decline in motor function, then psychiatric medications (antidepressants, anxiolytics, or even antipsychotics) may be needed to curb the abnormally increased sexual desire.

Medications for Seborrheic Dermatitis and Blepharitis

Hydrocortisone cream, dandruff shampoo, and ketoconazole (brand name Nizoral), a local medication used to treat fungal infections of the skin, are helpful in treating oiliness and flakiness of the skin of the face, eyebrows, and scalp. When the condition spreads to the eyelids (blepharitis), inflammation can be treated with wet, warm compresses (a simple alternative is a warm, wet teabag). Artificial tears may be needed to prevent the inflammation from becoming an infection and spreading to the eye itself. In more severe cases, a dermatologist or ophthalmologist should be consulted.

Brain Surgery for Parkinson's Disease

A Little History and an Overview

It may come as a surprise to learn that brain surgery has been effective in treating the symptoms of Parkinson's disease for more than 70 years. Brain surgery for Parkinson's started in the 1930s after physicians noticed that some people with a Parkinson's-related tremor were suddenly tremor free after having small strokes. **Neurosurgeons** and neurologists thought that if they could induce a small, controlled stroke or other similar small lesion in certain parts of the brain, they might be able to improve many of the symptoms that make life difficult for people with Parkinson's disease. In those early years, no effective medications were available for Parkinson's, so many people with the disease agreed to the surgery—this despite the fact that the success rate of these early procedures was very low, while the rate of serious complications was very high.

> **Brain surgery** has been a risky and variably effective treatment for Parkinson's disease for more than 80 years; however, scientific and technological advances of the last 30 years have turned brain surgery into a very effective treatment for some patients.

The rationale behind this brain surgery was that the symptoms of Parkinson's stem from an imbalance in the electrical activity of certain brain structures that are charged with controlling movement. This theory is considered valid even today. Chapter 2 discussed how the brain, using dopamine, achieves movement control through a sort of "push-pull" mechanism. In Parkinson's disease, the lack of dopamine causes too little of the "pushing" or the "pulling" in some brain structures and too much of it in others. The result is that while some neurons become less active or even die, others end up working too much. By silencing these hyperactive neurons, brain surgery rebalances the system and helps control tremors, bradykinesia, and rigidity. This neurosurgical strategy is called **functional neurosurgery**. Early procedures achieved this result either by removing small parts of the brain cortex (the outside part of the brain hemispheres) or by cutting the connection between the brain and muscles by snipping nerve fibers in the spinal cord or the nerve roots as they come out of the spinal column. In the 1940s, the procedure that seemed to be most effective was snipping a bundle of fibers in the brain that connected two groups of neurons in the **basal ganglia** (the structure deep inside the brain that regulates movement). That procedure is called ansotomy.

> Pallidotomy, thalamotomy, and DBS are various forms of **functional neurosurgery** for Parkinson's disease.

At about the same time, in the late 1940s, a new approach to doing brain surgery was developed, called **stereotaxic surgery**. In this approach, a probe is lowered into the brain through a small hole in the skull, thereby minimizing the overall brain trauma of the surgery. The probe uses an electric current (heat or freezing may also be used) to make a small, controlled lesion, or hole, in the brain tissue surrounding the probe's tip. Detailed brain maps helped doctors calculate the exact track of the probe needed to reach the intended target. This way, neurosurgeons could induce small lesions in deep brain structures that could not possibly be reached with open-brain surgery (at least not without a high risk of major brain damage). Two new procedures using the stereotaxic technique became popular in the 1950s, called **pallidotomy** and **thalamotomy**. These names derive from the brain structure that was lesioned in each (the **globus pallidus**, or **pallidum**, and the **thalamus**, respectively). Although these procedures were sometimes successful, the equipment was not precise, resulting in some patients having strokes or bleeding in the brain. Also, the chance of putting a lesion in the wrong place was high. So, when levodopa appeared in the 1960s, these surgeries became nearly extinct.

In the late 1980s, doctors realized that levodopa was not quite as effective as it had been hoped in patients with advanced stages of Parkinson's disease. During the 30 years between the 1950s and 1980s, technology had made wonderful advances. The development of computers allowed for better imaging of the brain (imaging is a term that describes all the various types of brain scans), which, in turn, permitted the construction of better brain maps. Neurosurgeons could now connect the stereotaxic probe to computerized equipment that could instantly analyze the electrical activity of the neurons close to its tip, thereby providing very accurate information about whether the probe was indeed at the intended target. And, scientists had dramatically expanded their understanding of the relationships among the various parts of the basal ganglia, thereby helping them to pick better targets. Scientists also had figured out a new way to silence the hyperactive neurons by applying a low-intensity, high-frequency current, rather than by killing them with electricity, heat, or freezing. Therefore, if the surgery was not effective, at least the wrong brain part was not permanently damaged. All these factors helped minimize complications and maximize the effectiveness of functional neurosurgery for Parkinson's disease.

A procedure called DBS (the details of which are discussed further in this chapter) is now frequently used to treat the symptoms of Parkinson's disease and some of the complications of its treatment. Besides DBS, some other forms of functional neurosurgery avoid the necessity of drilling a hole through the skull by remotely inducing a small lesion in the appropriate basal ganglia structure with highly focused beams of radiation or ultrasound. Although these techniques may be preferred in people for whom anesthesia is very risky, they again work by inducing a small lesion in the brain, so any unwanted effects may not be reversible.

> Transplantation of adrenal, fetal, and stem cells are past and proposed forms of **restorative neurosurgery** for Parkinson's disease.

Besides functional neurosurgery, doctors have tried to use brain surgery to "cure" Parkinson's. If the reason people get the disease is a lack of dopamine-producing neurons in the substantia nigra, then why not implant dopamine-producing neurons? Wouldn't that fix the problem once and for all? Organ transplantation works for the liver, heart, and kidneys, so why not for brain cells? Surgery for Parkinson's disease with this goal is called **restorative neurosurgery**. Finding a restorative procedure that cures Parkinson's disease is one of the holy grails of modern medicine. The biggest challenge is where to find dopamine neurons to implant. Who is the donor? Unlike other cells of our body, neurons do not multiply. We are born with a certain number of neurons and lose some every day as we age. Other cells in our body get renewed constantly; our skin cells, blood cells, and the cells lining our stomach, mouth, and intestines keep multiplying throughout our life. The reason people can afford to donate a part of their liver is that the donated portion will grow back. Bone marrow transplants are possible because a very small amount of donated bone marrow cells is sufficient to replenish the entire bone marrow of the person receiving the transplant.

So, for transplantation of dopamine-producing cells to be possible, a source had to be found that didn't consist of neurons. In the 1980s, scientists tried using a type of cell from the adrenal glands as donor cells. These cells produce a chemical similar to dopamine called **adrenaline**, and the hope was that implanting these cells in the brain might provide more raw material from which the brain could make dopamine. Despite early excitement, a large study conducted in the United States did not show any evidence of a consistent benefit from these adrenal transplants, and the surgery was soon abandoned. Then doctors looked for a source of immature cells that were destined to become dopamine neurons. This led to transplantation of fetal cells, immature nerve cells obtained from the developing brains of human fetuses that had recently died because of miscarriage or selective abortion. Many ethical questions had to be settled before these studies could proceed. In addition, some of the people with Parkinson's who volunteered for the studies had to agree to undergo brain surgery without actually receiving a transplant. Such "sham operations" are necessary so that comparisons can be made between groups of patients who have undergone the exact same procedures except for the treatment under investigation.

The first study of fetal transplants was published in 2001. As a group, patients who received the transplant did not do better than the patients who had sham operations. However, when scientists separated the patients by age, they found that people younger than 60 years of age who had the transplant did better than those who had the sham procedure. Unfortunately, a few months to years after the surgery, some of the successful cases developed dyskinesia like those that occur after long-term treatment with levodopa. Although these patients were taking levodopa, their dyskinesia persisted even after levodopa was discontinued.

In recent years, enthusiasm about fetal transplants declined even further. One of the "successful" cases died, and scientists were able to look in this person's brain. They found an unpleasant surprise: Parkinson's disease had affected the transplanted cells as well. Nevertheless, a lot was learned from these studies. For one thing, scientists confirmed that grafted cells can survive, produce dopamine, and develop connections with other neurons. Second, in younger patients, measurable improvement was seen.

Thus, research is continuing, and now scientists are looking into another source of donor dopamine neurons: stem cells. Stem cells are immature cells that have the potential to develop into all kinds of highly specialized cells (as opposed to just neurons). Over the past decade, scientists have been increasing their understanding of the processes that take place for a stem cell to grow into, for example, a dopamine-producing neuron. The concept behind restorative neurosurgery with stem cells is that one could implant these cells into the basal ganglia, then coax them into becoming dopamine-producing neurons and developing all the necessary connections, thereby fixing the problem that's causing the disease. Although this sounds promising, the disappointing results of the previous restorative procedures have made scientists cautious about proceeding with experimentation on people before some fundamental questions are answered through animal experiments. Taking the scientific argument one step further, some researchers are asking what would keep whatever is killing a person's dopamine neurons in the first place from attacking the transplanted cells as well. In fact, the case of the patient mentioned previously who underwent fetal transplantation suggests such an attack may be likely.

It is not the purpose of this book to discuss the ethics of stem cell research beyond pointing out that the use of tissues derived from human fetuses remains highly controversial from a philosophical point of view and is morally highly objectionable to many people. This fact makes it even more imperative that the science proceeds cautiously and that our understanding of the biological and scientific issues is optimized before we can talk about human experimentation.

> **Deep brain stimulation** works by resetting the balance of the electrical activity of brain structures involved in the control of voluntary movements.

Deep Brain Stimulation

The most commonly used brain surgery for Parkinson's disease is DBS. In DBS surgery, the surgeon inserts a wire (similar to a pacemaker wire) in a certain brain structure (the structure is discussed in material that follows). Each side of the brain controls the opposite side of the body. So, if the symptoms are really bad on the right and quite mild on the left, inserting the wire in the left side of the brain may be sufficient. When the wire is inserted only in one side of the brain, it is called a unilateral procedure. Most people with Parkinson's who benefit from this surgery will end up needing a wire on both sides (a bilateral procedure). Some neurosurgeons prefer to do a bilateral procedure in one session rather than two separate procedures. The wire is placed in its intended position (the target) through a burr hole in the skull, usually an inch or two to the side of and a little forward of the crown. The wire (or wires, for bilateral procedures) is then connected to a battery pack, which is implanted under the skin of the patient's chest, just as with a heart pacemaker. This unit is called the **neurotransmitter** (not to be confused with the chemical neurotransmitters that send signals between neurons). The stimulation can be turned on or off or be adjusted from the outside with a magnet and a specialized computer.

As mentioned, in Parkinson's disease, some neurons deep inside the brain in the basal ganglia become hyperactive from the loss of dopamine. The external stimulation from the deep brain stimulator silences or suppresses these neurons and in this way resets the balance of the push-pull function of the basal ganglia. Such overactive neurons can be found in a structure very close to the substantia nigra, called the **subthalamic nucleus,** as well as in the pallidum and the thalamus. The neurologist and neurosurgeon choose one of these three structures to target for DBS depending on the symptoms they hope to alleviate. Most people with Parkinson's who undergo this kind of surgery currently get subthalamic or pallidal stimulation. Thalamic stimulation is reserved for patients in whom tremor is the overwhelming problem, without much trouble from other symptoms.

In general terms, symptoms that seem to respond better to DBS are tremors, dyskinesia, and motor fluctuations (or wearing off). In fact, studies showed that people who have DBS to improve their symptom control during the day experience an average of 6 hours less "off" times during any given the day as a result. This is quite a bit better than can be achieved through medication adjustments. Symptoms that are not likely to improve and may even get worse because of the surgery are speech, balance trouble, and cognitive difficulties or dementia.

The Ask the Experts box discusses further details of DBS surgery for Parkinson's disease and provides information on who should be considered a good candidate, what reasonable expectations for the surgery are, how to weigh its pros and cons, and a little about the logistics.

Ask the Experts: Should I Have DBS Surgery?
What's Involved?

*Sierra Farris, PA-C, MPAS, gives us an overview of DBS:
"Medications that treat the motor symptoms of Parkinson's disease can be effective for many years. But, over time, many patients experience a 'wearing-off' effect. Many people also eventually experience dyskinesia or involuntary movements. These changes over time can be disruptive to a person's life. One way to minimize or eliminate the wearing-off effect and dyskinesia is by a treatment called deep brain stimulation (DBS). DBS is a surgical treatment option for patients who continue to have medication-responsive symptoms. Although brain surgery may sound scary, DBS has improved the lives of thousands of people living with Parkinson's, but it does come with the risks of having surgery.*

"Here's how it works: Parkinson's disease results from diminishing dopamine in the brain, and DBS compensates for the lack of dopamine by stimulating specific areas of the brain with electrical impulses. These microbursts of energy are focused in the globus pallidus internus or the subthalamic nucleus. These areas of the brain send signals that coordinate and control movements.

"The surgical procedure is separated into two stages. In the first operation, a surgeon inserts a DBS lead wire into the brain target after confirming that the location is satisfactory by testing the patient's response to stimulation while awake. This complex, detailed surgery takes several hours. In the second surgery, a neurotransmitter is implanted under the skin, typically in the upper chest area. The neurotransmitter is connected to an extension wire, which is connected to the lead wire. The neurotransmitter is similar in size to a cardiac pacemaker, and, like a pacemaker, the neurotransmitter provides constant electrical stimulation to its target. In the case of DBS, the stimulation mimics the effects of medication once the neurostimulator is set to optimal or therapeutic settings.

"*After the surgeries are complete and the neurotransmitter is operating at optimal settings—this must be achieved gradually over a period of weeks or months—most patients experience several benefits. One benefit is a significant reduction or complete elimination of the wearing-off effect. Patients using DBS therapy experience much more 'on' time. Another benefit is significant reduction in involuntary movements. And the third benefit, much desired by most patients, is a decrease in the amount of medication needed—many patients end up taking smaller and less frequent doses of drugs.*

"*A 2006 European study of 156 patients with severe motor complications of Parkinson's disease found that 'patients in the DBS group experienced a 25 percent average improvement in quality of life scores and a 41 percent average improvement in motor function' compared with 'no change on either measure among those patients in the non-DBS group.' The study was published in the* New England Journal of Medicine.

"*It's important to note that DBS does not cure Parkinson's disease. In addition, DBS is not a good treatment for gait freezing, falls, or speech problems. Symptoms that do not respond well to medication won't be helped by DBS. The surgery does not come without risks, including bleeding in the brain, infection, and, infrequently, misplaced wires requiring additional surgery.*

"*Patients who might be good candidates for DBS are those who can answer true to the following statements:*

- "*Levodopa still helps control the movement symptoms of Parkinson's disease.*
- "*My medicine doesn't last from dose to dose or wears off before the next dose is due.*
- "*My medicine still works but isn't controlling my tremor.*
- "*Dyskinesia is limiting my activities, is bothersome, or is causing pain.*
- "*My mind is still sharp, and I am not having hallucinations.*

- *"My mood is not depressed or anxious.*
- *"I don't mind living with an implanted device in my brain or body.*
- *"My family is supportive, and I can travel for DBS appointments as necessary.*

"After the DBS surgeries, there are few restrictions other than realizing that the DBS device is composed of wires that can be broken as a result of an accident. Patients must also avoid arc-welding equipment and strong electromagnetic fields. Some medical procedures are not permitted for patients who have had DBS, including body MRIs [magnetic resonance imaging] and therapeutic ultrasound such as diathermy, because of danger of stroke, coma, or death.

"People with joint problems or who may need an MRI should talk to their doctor about getting the MRI before DBS surgery. Some MRIs may be performed in people who have had DBS, but only with specialized equipment that's not widely available. Medtronic—the company that manufactures current DBS devices—has customer and technical patient services to answer questions that your healthcare providers may have about safety issues related to radiology, testing procedures, and surgery in people with DBS.

"Here are questions to ask your neurologist about DBS:

- *"What do you think will improve for me after surgery?*
- *"Who will program or determine the stimulation settings for me? (Programming the DBS neurotransmitter requires a skilled, licensed medical professional.)*
- *"How many other patients are you seeing who have one of these devices, and how have they improved with DBS?*

"Here are several questions to ask a surgeon about DBS:
- *"Is DBS the focus of your practice?*
- *"How many people have you implanted?*
- *"Who should I call if I have a problem after I leave the hospital?*
- *"What is your experience with complications from the surgery?"*

The Future of Surgery for Parkinson's Disease

Deep brain stimulation is not the last word on surgery for Parkinson's disease. In fact, in this chapter we touched only on the "hot issues" in Parkinson's surgery. But medicine usually evolves in many different directions simultaneously, and there is no telling which path will lead to the next major breakthrough. Although DBS has been very helpful for a group of people with certain complications of the disease, scientists are still working on finding better targets in the brain where DBS may be beneficial for symptoms not improved by the currently available procedures. Scientists also are trying to find other ways of using brain surgery to cure the disease. It is beyond the scope of this book to discuss the avenues of research that look promising today because this information changes rapidly, even as the ink on these pages is drying. New techniques may make use of genetically modified cells or viruses to restore brain chemistry and rebalance neuronal activity. For now, it is enough to remember that every small step counts, and that, despite not having reached the goal of curing Parkinson's disease, the surgical approach to treating it has been a source of otherwise unobtainable knowledge that has dramatically improved our understanding of the disease. Surgery is expected to continue to be a powerful research and treatment tool.

CHAPTER 8

Disease Management

Rehabilitation Therapy, Assistive Devices, and Adaptive Equipment

In this chapter, you will learn about

- How physical, occupational, and speech therapy can help manage the symptoms of Parkinson's
- Which assistive devices and adaptive equipment can help improve activities of daily living, and balance and prevent falls
- When, where, and how to look for assistive devices and adaptive equipment

In this chapter, we focus on the important role of the rehabilitation team in providing help and assistance for patients and caregivers. Although medications play a primary role in helping to manage many of the symptoms of Parkinson's disease, growing evidence indicates that rehabilitation therapies are important to the overall care plan. As care needs change, many patients seek guidance from physical, occupational, or speech therapists at various times in their journey with Parkinson's. These rehabilitation specialists are trained to help patients improve or maintain functional movement, communication, and involvement in daily life so the patients can reach their fullest potential.

This chapter also offers advice on devices and equipment that can make life easier for people with Parkinson's disease.

Physical Therapy

Scientific research shows that physical therapy helps patients with Parkinson's when added to a standard regimen of medication. Physical therapists are trained professionals who work to improve or restore mobility in their patients while providing ongoing education to ensure patients' understanding and follow-through. Recent laboratory studies have shown that physical exercise may benefit brain function by helping remaining dopamine work more efficiently. These studies also seem to suggest that the early addition of physical exercise to Parkinson's treatment provides the greatest benefit. Thus, it is important to seek physical therapy evaluation and treatment even in the early stages of Parkinson's disease to ensure that an appropriate exercise program is added to your daily routine.

Parkinson's disease causes changes in both mobility and perception. People with Parkinson's tend to make slower and smaller motions when walking, bending, or reaching than people without the disease. This smallness of movement, referred to as **hypokinesia**, affects most functional movements and can contribute to shuffling gait, loss of arm swing, and feelings of fatigue. As the motions become smaller, perception is also affected, so that people with Parkinson's begin to feel that these smaller motions are of normal size. Focused attention and practicing larger, exaggerated motions (often known as the **LSVT BIG** protocol) can be helpful in "recalibrating" the brain to achieve full, normal-size movements. People with Parkinson's often benefit from deliberately making their motions "too big" to compensate for hypokinesia. Working with a physical therapist on exercises, walking, and functional activities focused on increasing movement size has proven beneficial for many patients.

> Deliberately making "big" movements is one technique that helps reduce the hypokinesia caused by Parkinson's.

The series of motions required to rise from a chair or get into and out of bed are learned sequences that we tend to perform without conscious thought. Parkinson's disease, however, causes difficulty in activating sequences of movement we usually place "on automatic." When the sequence is difficult to activate, these once-simple tasks become increasingly difficult. Physical therapists can help patients perform such tasks by breaking down the sequence and working on each step in the process until it becomes easier.

Parkinson's-related muscle stiffness and rigidity have potential long-term complications, including loss of flexibility, reduction in muscle strength, changes in posture, and pain. Physical therapists can recommend stretching exercises and techniques for postural alignment and pain control. Relaxation training may also be used to help reduce stress and muscle tension.

Many patients begin to notice balance changes after living with Parkinson's disease for some time. Balance changes may vary with each individual and can present as freezing, backward loss of balance (also called retropulsion), difficulty turning corners, or falling. A physical therapist can assess balance difficulties and offer instruction on appropriate exercises, balance safety strategies, assistive walking devices to improve safety and reduce fall risk, or some combination of these approaches. If a patient is injured in a fall, physical therapists can work in hospital, transitional care, home care, and outpatient settings to help the individual return to his or her preinjury level of function.

Occupational Therapy

Although the word *occupational* might make one think that an occupational therapist helps with on-the-job skills, this skilled professional actually does much more. In truth, occupational therapists help patients better perform numerous kinds of daily tasks. Each person's daily routine is unique, but it usually includes self-care activities such as dressing, bathing, brushing teeth, and combing hair. Many people are involved in household chores that may include cooking, laundry, housekeeping, and yard work. We also tend to drive cars, maintain our finances, manage medication schedules, and do other tasks requiring concentration, memory, handwriting, or typing. Daily life can involve not only a regular work schedule but also usually some pursuit of leisure interests and hobbies. Occupational therapists play a role in helping those with Parkinson's perform all these activities.

A thorough assessment by an occupational therapist will usually include a comprehensive evaluation of arm and hand function, including flexibility, strength, and coordination. The therapist may recommend exercises to improve or maintain function of the upper extremities or may recommend adaptive equipment that allows the person with Parkinson's disease to perform a daily task with greater ease.

Task analysis of activities performed in the daily routine will often result in recommendations to improve the ease and safety of such regular activities. For example, an occupational therapist may assess the risk of falling and provide recommendations to reduce this risk as a person moves around the kitchen to prepare a meal or may offer suggestions for installation of bathroom safety equipment to ensure safe bathing and toileting. Some occupational therapists are involved in evaluating worksites to suggest ways to enhance and improve performance of job tasks, while others offer in-depth assessments of safety and vehicle operation while a person is driving.

Occupational therapists also offer assessment of and insight into visual, perceptual, or cognitive changes caused by Parkinson's disease. If deficits are identified, occupational therapists work with a patient and the patient's family to offer recommendations to lessen or compensate for these deficits. Examples include suggestions to make reading easier or developing a system to keep medications on schedule. An occupational therapy referral may also be helpful for obtaining recommendations for modifying performance of leisure activities and hobbies or to offer suggestions for new areas of interest.

If Parkinson's disease results in a significant loss of mobility, occupational therapists are often involved in the assessment and fitting of appropriate wheelchair and seating systems to ensure good positioning and comfort and prevent skin breakdown. Education of family members and care partners also becomes important if the person with Parkinson's requires more hands-on assistance to perform daily self-care tasks.

Speech Therapy

An estimated 98 percent of people with Parkinson's disease experience changes in communication. Speech pathologists are professionals who specialize in the treatment of speech and language disorders. Research shows that speech therapy treatment can reduce the communication deficits caused by Parkinson's disease.

Changes to the motor and sensory processing systems can affect communication. Many people with Parkinson's disease are frustrated by frequent requests to repeat themselves during conversation. Patients often develop a condition referred to as hypokinetic dysarthria, in which the slowed, smaller motions of people with Parkinson's disease affect muscles in the face, lips, and tongue used to produce speech. There can also be smallness of movement in the respiratory system, which provides breath support to produce voice volume. These movement changes result in soft, slurred speech that is often difficult to understand.

Changes in sensory processing can cause people with Parkinson's disease to feel they are speaking in a normal audible voice when, in fact, their speech is soft and difficult to hear. Such individuals often need to exert an effort that feels like shouting to achieve a normal speaking voice. Speech therapy techniques can help them to recalibrate their voices to turn up the volume and speak appropriately loudly on a consistent basis. Specially trained speech pathologists use a technique called **LSVT–LOUD**, which is based on clinical research, to maximize voice volume in individuals with Parkinson's disease.

Speech pathologists also provide comprehensive evaluation and treatment for people experiencing dysphagia, or difficulty swallowing. The speech pathologist will assess swallowing through evaluation of musculature and a review of the person's posture and positioning when eating. Special tests such as a **video swallowing assessment** (a kind of x-ray of the swallowing mechanism) may also be recommended. Treatment may include exercises to improve the swallowing mechanism, recommendations for improved posture and positioning at mealtime, and suggestions for diet modification. The speech pathologist will also discuss and address excessive salivation and techniques to minimize drooling.

For people experiencing changes in memory, concentration, or thought processes, a speech pathologist may become involved in overall assessment and treatment to improve these cognitive deficits or provide compensation strategies. As Parkinson's disease progresses, communication may become more difficult and more important, because patients with Parkinson's have to be able to communicate about their needs or discomfort. Communication may develop into a source of frustration for both patients and care partners. At this stage, referrals to speech therapy often focus on designing alternative forms of communication or the use of specialized communication assistive devices.

Assistive Devices and Adaptive Equipment

A variety of useful tools and equipment can make living with Parkinson's disease easier. Seeking out this equipment can be somewhat daunting because literally thousands of pieces of equipment are available in stores and catalogs or on websites. It is often helpful to speak with members of your healthcare team before making an equipment purchase, as they have more experience and will be able to provide you with recommendations to ensure that you obtain items that will be useful at the lowest possible expense.

Some equipment (e.g., gait-assistive devices like canes and walkers) may be covered by medical insurance. But choose wisely: a hasty purchase may prove to be a costly mistake. Many insurance plans will only cover one such device every 5 years, so before purchasing such equipment, make sure you have reviewed the options carefully and have obtained recommendations from your team, who can offer suggestions and instruction in proper use. Other types of equipment (including adapted silverware, shower benches, and kitchen utensils) are usually *not* covered by insurance. It is easy to order the wrong item because there are many varieties. Make sure your purchase is designed to do what you are hoping it will and seek recommendations from your team or from others with Parkinson's disease who have experience using that specific item.

Next, we provide answers to many commonly asked questions related to equipment that will make living with Parkinson's disease easier.

Where Should Grab Bars Be Installed?

The most important equipment is items that make living in your home safer. Most people living with Parkinson's disease would benefit from the installation of safety grab bars in their bathroom near the shower, tub, and toilet. Make sure that these items are installed correctly and securely into the studs of the wall. When moving around the bathroom, avoid using grab bar substitutes, such as soap dishes, faucet handles, and shower rods. These items can easily come off the wall if too much pressure is applied to them, and you could be injured.

In addition to these bathroom modifications, some people have found it beneficial to install a vertical grab bar next to the door of their home either on the inside or on the outside (whichever side the door pulls open from). This provides a sturdy hold and can reduce the risk of backward loss of balance when pulling the door open.

What About Stair Railings?

Stair railings should be installed in all indoor and outdoor stairways in the home. When possible, railings should be installed on both sides of the stairs. Make sure railings extend the entire length of the staircase. If the original railing is too short, you may need to add an additional length of railing. In some homes, it may be possible to extend the railing up onto the wall at the top of the stairs. This helps prevent the individual with Parkinson's from bending or stooping excessively to reach down to the rail when descending from the top.

If the person needs support when walking, railings can also be installed in hallways or the bedroom. An accessible ramp may work best for steps into the garage or outdoors.

What Other Types of Equipment Help Promote Bathroom Safety?

Standing in the shower or climbing into a bathtub may prove difficult or unsafe for those with balance changes related to Parkinson's disease. Consider purchasing a sturdy shower or tub bench. These items come in several styles. Obtaining a bench with a backrest is often recommended because it reduces the risk of backward balance loss. Some styles of benches bridge over the side of the tub, allowing the user to first sit down on the outside of the tub before sliding her or his legs across for bathing.

If balance changes require you to take a seated shower, consider buying a simple handheld showerhead, which is easy for most people to use and spray where they want. If you feel safe enough to take a shower standing, be sure to use nonskid strips or a mat in the bottom of the tub.

If rising from a seated position is proving more difficult, an elevated toilet seat may make doing so easier and safer. You can have a higher toilet installed if you are considering renovations or can purchase an elevated seat that can be clamped onto the existing toilet. Avoid molded plastic seats that do not clamp firmly to the sides of the toilet. Some elevated seats have attached armrests for added support, while others require installing a grab bar on the adjoining wall.

You can use a small bench or chair with a backrest next to the bathroom sink when shaving, brushing your teeth, applying makeup, or doing other tasks normally done from a standing position. People who experience frequent backward balance loss will definitely benefit from this adaptation.

Are There Any Other Tips for Bathroom Safety?

- Using "soap on a rope" or installing a body wash dispenser on the wall prevents having to bend forward to search for dropped soap in the bottom of the tub or shower.
- Some people with Parkinson's find it difficult to dry off after bathing, as muscle rigidity may make it difficult to reach one's back. Don a fluffy terrycloth robe to help absorb moisture and dry off quickly.
- Taped lines in the doorway threshold or a taped X in front of the sink or toilet serves as a visual cue to aid people who have freezing episodes in a small, enclosed bathroom space.
- Make sure lighting is adequate for nighttime trips to the bathroom. Darkened or shadowy rooms promote balance loss and freezing.

How Can I Stay Safer in the Kitchen?

Moving between the counter, stove, sink, table, and refrigerator while preparing food requires frequent stops, starts, and turns. Be mindful of trying to turn corners in a wide arc when moving away from the counter or sink. Place one hand on the counter or shelf when reaching overhead to get items from the cupboard. Consider rearranging your kitchen to place the most commonly used items on the lowest shelf or on the counter. Avoid using step stools to reach into high cabinets.

A number of adaptive cutting boards and knives are available to make food preparation easier. Always make sure you are using good potholders or oven mitts when cooking on the stove or reaching into the oven. Consider obtaining a kitchen stool or chair to sit on while cooking; this may help you maintain balance. If reaching into the oven becomes too difficult, use a microwave or toaster oven.

Consider buying covered cups and nonglass dishes instead of glass dishes. Practice sliding dishes along the counter or use a small kitchen cart to avoid carrying a lot of things in your hands. (Remember that multitasking becomes difficult with Parkinson's disease and sometimes leads to balance loss or falls.) Work with the occupational therapist on your team to solve specific difficulties you encounter in your own kitchen.

I Am Having Difficulty Rising from a Chair. Would a Lift Chair Work for Me?

Chairs with an electric-lift component slowly raise a person from a seated to a near-standing position. In many cases, this is an appropriate option to ensure safety and independence. While some people are concerned that they may become dependent on the chair, it does not have to be used consistently. However, it can be very useful when one needs to get up quickly (as when answering the door or the telephone). An electric-lift chair may also be good for people experiencing motor fluctuations that result in difficulty rising at some times but not others.

Medical equipment companies and some furniture stores carry electric-lift reclining chairs. They come in a variety of shapes and sizes. If possible, go to the store and try sitting in the chair to assess its comfort and how it suits your posture before purchase.

Some medical insurance plans provide a stipend for purchasing electric-lift chairs if the patient has a letter of medical necessity. Check with your plan to find out if this is an option for you and what information needs to be submitted before purchase. If your insurance does not help pay for the chair and finances are an issue, consider buying a used chair advertised in the classified section of a newspaper or online.

Is There Equipment to Make Mobility at Night or in Bed Easier?

Many people with Parkinson's have difficulty turning in bed at night because muscle rigidity and slowness affect their legs, arms, and trunk. The reduction in medication over the nighttime hours may also make moving in bed more difficult. Simple strategies such as using a satin-based fabric through the middle third of the bed or wearing silk or acetate fabric nightwear make rolling easier. Full satin sheets, however, are often too slippery, offering poor foot traction on the bed.

For some people, a half side rail or bed pole provides a sturdy grip and makes getting in and out of bed easier. Make sure any device you use is attached firmly and will support your weight during the position change. Avoid half side rails that are too long, preventing you from easily getting your hips in and out of bed. Overhead bed trapezes often do not work well because they do not allow you sufficient leverage to get your legs moving. It should be noted that some senior residential communities and nursing homes do not allow the use of certain types of bed mobility assistive equipment. If you or your loved one lives in this type of care setting, you may want to check with the care staff regarding guidelines for use for purchasing and using this type of equipment.

Good lighting is essential when getting up at night. Shadows or darkened rooms create the potential for balance loss and falls. Consider having an easily accessible lamp or a motion-detecting nightlight if you do not like to have lights on while sleeping

Some people with Parkinson's experience the frequent need or urge to urinate at night, resulting in multiple hurried trips to the bathroom. Consider buying a bedside urinal or commode to make this need easier to accommodate.

Do I Need a Hospital Bed?

Hospital beds are usually used only by people with significant mobility problems who need special assistance with transfers and bed mobility. These beds usually come with side rails. Some beds are electric and have a remote control to adjust the bed height or to raise the head or foot of the bed (or both). Other beds have a manual crank mechanism to make these adjustments. Check with your insurance plan to see what type of bed it may cover. (Figure 8.1 shows a hospital bed with some useful features.) Foam mattress pads or electric alternating-pressure pads for hospital beds can be obtained for people with severe mobility problems and the potential for skin breakdown. Retail stores and online sellers also offer beds that are not hospital beds but have mechanisms for adjusting the bed into a number of positions.

Is There Equipment to Make Getting Into and Out of the Car Easier?

Satin-based fabric or a cushion may make it easier to slide into and out of a car. A small tool called a Handybar can also help; it fits into the door latch on most cars to create a hand rest one can use when rising. Some people have used a suction-grip grab bar on the top of the car as an added way to stabilize themselves during the transfer.

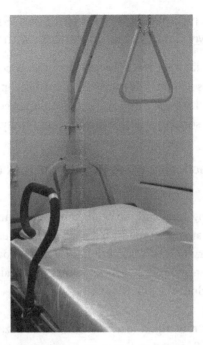

FIGURE 8.1 Aids for mobility in bed. A hospital bed has controls for raising the head or foot of the bed. Patients with Parkinson's find the type of rail attachment shown at lower left easier to use than the standard bedrails that come with a hospital bed. The bright tape provides a visual cue that may be especially important if a person's vision is affected. Bedclothes of satin or similar slippery fabric improve mobility in bed. This bed has a trapeze overhead, which is not always very helpful to people with Parkinson's.

If you're considering purchasing a new car, don't buy one with low seats that make rising more difficult. Choose leather or vinyl over cloth seats, which often make it more difficult to scoot over. Seats with built-in lumbar support may also help with posture and positioning when riding.

If you use a wheelchair at all times, you can get a van fitted with an electric lift that allows you to be transported in the chair.

A physical therapist or occupational therapist can work with you to make car transfers safer and easier.

What Do I Do If Car Transfers Do Not Seem Safe or Feasible for My Care Partner to Perform with Me?

Investigate special transportation services in your community. Most of these services will provide transport to medical appointments and other events with advance notice and scheduling. Fees vary based on the vendor and services available in your community.

Are There Practical Ways to Reduce the Risk of Injury from Falling?

If you are falling frequently in your home environment, it may be helpful to look at your home with a fresh eye and remove items that may cause injury in a fall. Obtaining knee and elbow pads for joint protection may also prove beneficial. Other practical suggestions for home safety include the following:

- Remove throw rugs, the most common fall hazard.
- Get rid of floor clutter that may contribute to tripping. Plant stands, footstools, magazine racks, and other low objects can all be hazardous.
- Rearrange furniture to create wide walking paths. Removing the coffee table from the center of the room can open up the space and reduce the risk of falls.
- Reduce the temptation to climb by removing footstools and ladders.
- Install vertical grab bars next to doors that pull toward you to minimize the risk of backward balance loss.
- Add lighting to ensure safe nighttime trips to the bathroom.
- Wear shoes with good support, low heels, and nonslip soles.
- Make sure your tub or shower has a nonslip mat.
- Avoid stepping over sleeping pets. Make sure your dog or cat is not underfoot before beginning to move.

How Much Should I Invest in Modifying My Home?

Home renovation or modifications can be time consuming and expensive. Before undertaking a major remodeling project, ask yourself a few questions. How long do I plan to stay in my current home? Will the modifications I make allow me to continue to live here? Do I have the financial resources to complete the renovation project? If you decide to start the remodeling project (or if you are moving to a new space and have choices in the finishing process), consider the following:

- Low-pile carpeting without excessive patterns or wood or laminate flooring is usually best for safe walking if you plan to use an assistive device or wheelchair.
- Make doorways wider if you use an assistive device or wheelchair or may need to do so in the future.
- Walk-in showers allow one to bathe without having to step over the edge of a tub.
- Shower curtains often are easier to move around than solid shower doors.
- Elevated toilets make transfer easier.
- Wide walking paths throughout the residence, without tight corners or excessive furniture, make mobility easier.
- Ramps may be installed in place of stairways, or electric stair glides may be installed to enable one to negotiate stairs safely.
- When possible, create one-level living, having the bedroom, bathroom, and living space all on one floor.
- A ramp or one-level living can make it easier to access the outdoors.
- Have a place where a care partner or live-in assistant can sleep within easy access or hearing distance of the person with Parkinson's if needed.

What Assistive Device Can Make My Walking Safer?

There are a variety of gait-assistive devices designed to promote safe walking and minimize loss of balance. It is highly recommended that you seek input from a physical therapist before purchasing such a device. Doing so will help ensure that you receive the most appropriate device, that it is adjusted to an appropriate height, and that you have received instructions in its proper use.

What Assistive Devices Do *Not* Typically Work Well for People with Parkinson's Disease?

Generally, any assistive device that interrupts the normal flow of walking may hinder someone with Parkinson's disease. Since people with Parkinson's typically walk with short, shuffling steps and have difficulty starting and stopping, devices like standard four-post walkers and quad canes (canes with a four-legged base) do not work well. Many people with Parkinson's who attempt to use these devices tend to carry them along without setting the legs firmly on the ground. This does not enhance walking stability and may actually promote loss of balance. Although well-meaning friends and family may try to loan you these devices, avoid using them. It's best to ask a physical therapist what device is best for you.

So, What Device May Best Aid My Walking?

Someone experiencing mild balance imprecision when walking or feelings of balance loss on uneven terrain may benefit from the use of a single-end cane or walking stick. These assistive devices do not interrupt the normal flow of walking, and their tips can be set down on the ground to widen the base of support, minimizing loss of balance.

Canes should be adjusted to allow 15–30 degrees of bend at the elbow when one is gripping the cane. When walking, the cane should be set firmly on the ground and not carried. A patient can work with a physical therapist to learn proper technique.

Many people have found that aluminum or wood walking sticks, also known as Nordic walking poles or hiking poles, provide balance support while enabling more upright posture. They are particularly helpful when one is walking on uneven terrain (for example, on grass, gravel, or uneven sidewalks). For best stability, one or two poles may be used. Hiking poles can usually be found at sporting goods stores. Again, seek instruction from a physical therapist for proper fitting and best use.

If a person needs additional walking support, a wheeled walker typically works best. Aluminum walkers with straight wheels on the front often are difficult to turn and may not offer adequate stability for longer distances or when outdoors. Consider adding swivel casters (the 5-inch size typically works best) to make turning safer with these devices. Glide brakes can also be added to allow safer stops.

Most people who require a walker find that one with four large wheels, swivel casters, hand brakes, and a bench seat (as shown on the left side of Figure 8.2) offers the greatest stability. Walkers like this easily move and turn. Make sure to choose a walker with a sturdy

FIGURE 8.2 Gait-assistive devices. Left: Four-wheel walker with hand brakes, carrying basket, and bench seat. Right: U-Step Walking Stabilizer.

frame and good brakes. Tall individuals or those with large frames may require specially designed heavy-duty metal walkers. The bench seat can double as a tray space to carry items while walking, and most walkers of this style also come with a basket or bag for other items. If you fatigue easily or have dizziness or fainting spells, the attached seat may be extremely useful, allowing you to sit down when needed.

There is a specialty walker designed specifically for those with movement disorders such as Parkinson's disease. The U-Step Walking Stabilizer (shown on the right side of Figure 8.2) has a heavy, very sturdy frame with multiple casters on a U-shaped base. It also has a "reverse brake" mechanism, meaning that it stays in a locked position until the user releases it by squeezing the hand brake. Tension can be added to the walker to reduce the speed of the device, which may be most helpful to individuals who experience bursts of speed when walking.

It is important to consider the portability of any assistive device. Some walkers are significantly heavier than others and may be difficult to lift into the trunk or back seat of a car. It is advisable to practice folding and lifting any assistive device before purchase to ensure that the person with Parkinson's or a family caregiver can safely lift and handle the device for transport.

Consult a physical therapist familiar with all these gait-assistive devices to help you select the right one and ensure that it is adjusted and used properly.

When Should I Consider Using a Wheelchair?

Wheelchairs are rarely needed in the early and moderate stages of Parkinson's disease. Use of a wheelchair is usually considered if mobility problems are preventing an individual from fully participating in home or community activities. While making the decision to use a wheelchair is often difficult, it is important to recognize that limiting one's activities is isolating, has a negative impact on quality of life, and may actually compromise independence and safety.

Some people choose to use a wheelchair only for going longer distances, attending social events, or shopping. In these cases, the wheelchair can help in combating fatigue and allow the person to become more fully engaged in the activity. Obtaining a lightweight transport chair that can be easily lifted into and out of the trunk of a car may work best for these situations.

If balance and mobility are more severely challenged, it may be necessary to obtain a wheelchair for more consistent use. When choosing a wheelchair, it is important to work with a physical therapist, occupational therapist, or vendor who has expertise in the options available and is trained in appropriate fitting. Options such as reclining chair backs, removable leg rests and armrests, brake extenders, seating cushions, and trunk supports should all be considered before a wheelchair purchase. Make sure the vendor provides information about and support for repair and maintenance of the chair.

The care partner should also have input to ensure the chair will fit within the home environment and can be disassembled and lifted safely into and out of the trunk of a car or van.

Can I Use an Electric Wheelchair or Scooter?

Many people think that the use of an electric device will solve their mobility problems. All too often, they are disappointed after a hastily made purchase. Electric wheelchairs and scooters are very heavy and may not be able to be broken down for transport, so that a van with an electric lift is necessary. These devices are also quite large and may not be able to be maneuvered safely at home. Some senior apartment complexes prohibit use of electric scooters and wheelchairs because of potential safety risks to others.

It is important to recognize that Parkinson's disease causes not only physical but also cognitive and perceptual challenges that may prevent an individual from operating an electric device safely. Motor fluctuations, excessive dyskinesia, freezing, postural instability, and changes in thinking and memory can all contribute to unsafe operation of motorized devices. We strongly recommend that a person's abilities be evaluated by a physical or occupational therapist before the purchase of a wheelchair or scooter.

What Adaptations Can Make Eating Easier?

Changes in fine-motor coordination and tremor can cause difficulties in cutting food, bringing food from the plate to your mouth, or drinking from a cup. These difficulties can cause frustration and keep people from enjoying social outings at restaurants with friends and family. Some of these frustrations can be reduced by asking for a steak knife to make cutting easier or asking for meat to be cut in the kitchen before serving.

Adapted eating utensils can also make mealtime easier (Figure 8.3). Rocker knives allow you to cut food in a rocking motion, improving

FIGURE 8.3 Adapted eating utensils. Clockwise from upper left are a "nosey cup," plate guard, right-handed curved fork and spoon, rocker knife, and a left-handed curved spoon, all sitting on a nonslip mat.

ease and reducing stress. Large-handled utensils may make eating easier. Forks and spoons with curved handles make it easier to bring food to the mouth without spilling. Plate guards create a ledge on the plate for people who have difficulty loading food onto a fork or spoon. Before purchasing such utensils, talk to an occupational therapist about what options might work best for a particular situation or condition.

Covered cups are readily available and can reduce spills related to tremor. If you have difficulty tipping your head back to drink easily, try a "nosey cup," which has a dip in one side so that the nose doesn't block the cup.

Are There Devices That Can Help My Communication?

We live in a high-tech society that has created a number of computerized devices designed to enhance communication. Many of these devices are very expensive and may not offer the consistent performance desired for ongoing use. The individual using the communication device needs to have adequate perception, cognition, and, in some cases, hand coordination to use them efficiently. Consult with a speech pathologist familiar with voice-activated and other electronic communication devices before making a purchase.

If an electronic device does not appear to be the answer, the speech pathologist can help you to work with low-tech devices, such as word or letter boards, hand signals or gestures, or other strategies for ongoing communication between the patient and the care partner or others. Simple strategies such as facing each other when speaking or reducing distracting noise in the environment are often helpful as well.

I Am Having Difficulty Remembering to Take My Pills on a Regular Schedule. What Can Help Me?

It is essential for people with Parkinson's to take their medications on time. Multiple dosing throughout the day can sometimes make it

FIGURE 8.4 Devices for remembering to take pills on time. Clockwise from left are a timer-equipped pillbox, pill organizer, and alarm watch.

difficult to remember to take pills at the right time. **Figure 8.4** shows several devices that are useful for reminding one to take pills.

Putting pills into pill organizers designed for this purpose can help a person stay on track. These boxes can be purchased at most pharmacies. Look for a box that can accommodate the pills in your regular schedule for a full day. If you forget to take your pills even after setting up a pill organizer, a timer can provide a useful reminder. Some pillboxes have a built-in timer that can be set to regular intervals, creating a beeping or buzzing sound as a reminder that it is "pill time." Some people use an alarm watch that can be set for several times throughout the day. In place of a sound, some watches can create a vibrating sensation on your wrist, alerting you that it is pill time without creating a disturbance in your surroundings.

If you are unsure what system will work best for you, a nurse or occupational therapist can review the options and help you make the best choice.

What Adaptations Can Be Made to My Computer?

A number of adaptations can enhance computer use. Computers can be set up to minimize letter repetitions resulting from repeated keystrokes due to slowness or tremor. It is also possible to set up voice-activated typing on your computer. Larger keyboards and monitor screens may also make computer use easier. Check with your occupational therapist about referral sources for adapted-computer services in your area.

The Multidisciplinary Approach

Knowledge in medicine advances in many different ways. As more specialists from the various therapeutic disciplines started targeting the symptoms of Parkinson's, they developed a new understanding of the disease and much was learned through experience, only to be later confirmed through rigorous research. This has led to specialization within the various disciplines. Physical, occupational, and speech therapists may specialize in treating Parkinson's disease; this is greatly facilitated within dedicated Parkinson's centers. The exposure to many people with Parkinson's and their daily challenges has led to a better understanding of the ways to help problem-solve, with the therapists from different disciplines often working together to address a problem. Falling is a good example; the causes of falling may be many, from orthostatic drops in the blood pressure to reduced clearance when walking, which leads to tripping, freezing of gait, and loss of balance reflexes, and the list may go on and on. Through a concerted effort, the movement disorders specialist, nurse, physical therapist, and occupational therapist may arrive at a better understanding of the causes of falling and the ways to prevent it for each case. The physician and nurse may review and adjust the medications and habits of the person with Parkinson's, the physical therapist may assess and retrain his or her strength and balance, and the occupational therapist may review the circumstances of the fall and the activity and environment factors that may be modified to minimize risk. This has become known as the multidisciplinary model of care and has been increasingly implemented by dedicated Parkinson's centers across the world with remarkable effect on the quality of life of people with Parkinson's and their families. Many such centers are great resources, with educational, outreach, community engagement, exercise, and social activities, and strive to be there for people with Parkinson's and their families throughout their journey with Parkinson's.

Can Technology Help Me Manage My Parkinson's Symptoms?

An increasing number of apps are available that have been designed for individuals living with Parkinson's. Apps can be easily downloaded to a phone or tablet to incorporate into everyday use. Some of the apps are free, while others involve a nominal cost. Apps are available to help people with Parkinson's practice and improve communication, remind them to take their medications on time, provide exercise suggestions and track progress, and record/monitor symptoms to discuss during physician or physical/occupational therapy visits. At this time, there is no one manufacturer or clearinghouse for these apps, and not every app will work well for each individual. You are encouraged to explore and experiment with the available resources to see if an app would work well for you. Physical, occupational, or speech therapists may be able to offer app recommendations appropriate for your specific needs.

Everyone who lives with Parkinson's disease sooner or later finds out that their body functions differently at different times of the day or night. During a visit to the doctor's or therapist's office, the medication may be working really well, and a person with Parkinson's may stand up and walk with ease, only to experience more balance problems and falling later in the day, when his or her treating specialists are not around to watch what happens. Doctors and therapists are now starting to use what is called "wearable technology" to monitor how the bodies of people with Parkinson's function as they go through their day-to-day activities. Some devices may monitor for the presence of tremors, dyskinesia, or wearing off; others are capable of recording falls, and yet others are aimed at the nonmotor symptoms of Parkinson's, such as noting blood pressure fluctuations.

Other devices that use smart technology are being developed to help manage some of the symptoms of Parkinson's. For example, one device worn on the chest senses when the person wearing it is leaning forward too much and gives a feedback signal (a beep or a gentle jolt) to remind the person to stand up straighter. Another device hidden in the handle of a utensil senses tremor and generates a vibration calculated to cancel out the effect of the tremor. Such devices may work for some people and not for others, but it is useful to know they exist and, more important, are being refined, so that they can be useful to more and more people in the future.

CHAPTER 9

Disease Management

Specific Symptoms

In this chapter, you will learn about

- The options you have when trying to manage specific motor symptoms day to day
- The options you have when trying to manage specific nonmotor symptoms day to day

As mentioned in Chapters 3 and 4, people living with Parkinson's disease may have to deal with a great variety of symptoms over the years. Naturally, in the earliest stages of the disease, the focus is on the motor problems: tremor, slow movement, and muscle stiffness. Generally, these symptoms respond adequately to medications that replenish the missing dopamine or provide a good substitute for it. As the disease progresses, balance may become more of a challenge, or patients may experience motor complications in the form of dyskinesia or wearing off. Fine-tuning of pill doses and a more complicated medication regimen may provide relief, but it is usually at this stage that patients begin to realize that they have to learn to live with some symptoms and that they may have to pick their battles about which symptoms are most important to treat and which to leave alone. It is also at this stage, with the increasing complexity of the drug regimen, that more side effects may arise. As the disease spreads in the brain, new symptoms may appear, such as confusion, dementia, hallucinations, and falling.

Most of these challenges in the advanced stages of the disease are not dopamine related, and dopamine drugs not only are useless in dealing with them but also may even aggravate them. What's more, for many of these symptoms, available medications either are ineffective or may be contraindicated because they can dramatically worsen mobility when given to a person with Parkinson's.

Many of the symptoms in advanced Parkinson's disease do not respond to drugs that act on the dopamine system. In fact, such medications may aggravate a lot of these symptoms.

In this chapter, we discuss some of the challenging symptoms of Parkinson's disease from the earliest to the more advanced stages. Because medications have already been discussed in Chapter 7, the focus is not so much on medications but rather on how one can learn to live with, or manage, some of these challenges. Surprising to some, many of the symptoms for which we do not have a "magic pill" respond to therapy intervention. With compensatory techniques, one can learn how to overcome a specific challenge by relying on strengths or learning new ways to perform specific tasks. With restorative techniques, one can train to strengthen weaker areas. It may also come as a surprise to many that such strategies are very important and effective in disease management from the earliest stages. In fact, many specialists in the field of Parkinson's disease believe that early involvement with therapy and exercise can result in a strong foundation that will be helpful in the later stages of the disease.

In this chapter, we also discuss how to deal with special circumstances, such as what a person with Parkinson's disease should know about having elective surgery or what to expect when hospitalized for some other illness to anticipate situations that might otherwise create unpleasant surprises.

Managing Tremor, Bradykinesia, and Rigidity

Parkinson's symptoms can fluctuate throughout the day depending on medication levels, fatigue, stress levels, and sometimes unknown reasons. Consider medication schedules when planning your daily routine, opting to do more complex tasks at times when your medication is functioning at its best. Allow adequate time to accomplish tasks and avoid hurrying. Schedule breaks as needed; tasks that you accomplished easily in the past may need to be broken down into several shorter sessions with rest in between. Remember that feelings of stress may make symptoms such as tremor and slowness feel even worse. It is usually best to be proactive and plan ahead to avoid feeling rushed. Start to get ready for scheduled appointments and events well in advance of your departure time.

Small, cramped handwriting (micrographia) can create difficulty and added stress in the daily routine. Figure 9.1 shows several tools that can help with handwriting. It can be helpful to use a large-grip pen and slow down when writing, focusing on making large, exaggerated letters. Printing rather than using a cursive form of writing also sometimes helps. Some people find that lined paper helps provide a visual cue for keeping letter sizes larger. To avoid stress in public situations where handwriting is needed, it may be helpful to prefill forms or check blanks before standing in line or use a credit or debit card to make purchases. If tremor interferes with writing or other activities that require a steady hand, sometimes wearing a weighted wristband (available in stores selling exercise gear) can help.

Seek out tools and adaptive equipment to make life easier. Buttonhooks, Velcro closures, elastic shoelaces, long shoehorns, and reachers can make dressing less cumbersome (Figure 9.2). Jar openers, cutting boards, and other kitchen gadgets reduce frustrations during meal preparation. Large handles on forks, toothbrushes, combs, and other personal items often make them easier to use in the daily routine. (See Chapter 8 for more details on adaptive equipment.) Covered cups can help decrease spills caused by tremor. Use of a steak knife or adapted rocker knives can make cutting foods easier. Ask for meat to

FIGURE 9.1 Tools that can help with handwriting. From left to right are a "fat" pen, a pen with an added grip, and a specialty pen for a modified grip, all sitting on lined paper.

FIGURE 9.2 Clothing and devices that make dressing easier. At left and right, respectively, are a shirt and pants with fake buttons and Velcro closures. At the bottom are an elastic shoelace (left) and a buttonhook (right). At the top are a reacher and a long-grip shoehorn.

be precut in the kitchen when dining at a restaurant if this is an issue for you. An occupational therapist can help you sort through the array of adaptive equipment on the market and make recommendations on what is most appropriate to your situation.

Be aware that mobility may decline during the nighttime hours, when you are less likely to be taking medication. As discussed in Chapter 8, nightwear made of a slippery fabric or sheets with a satin-based fabric through the middle third of the bed can make rolling easier. Use adequate nighttime lighting for trips to the bathroom. Speak with your medical provider if you experience significant changes in nighttime mobility. Medication adjustments may help remedy this problem. Rehabilitation therapists can also teach safe and effective strategies to make bed mobility easier and can make recommendations for equipment such as a half side rail or bed pole as needed.

Change position frequently throughout the day to reduce feelings of stiffness and muscle rigidity. Try to do occasional stretches for your neck, shoulders, and trunk if you are sitting in a chair or at a desk or computer for long periods. Use of a lumbar support cushion in the chair or car can improve sitting posture and reduce back tension and stiffness. The "slippery fabric" concept can also work with getting in and out of a car. Some people find that putting a plastic bag (a trash bag works well) on the car seat reduces friction and makes it easier to swing the legs in and out of the car.

Managing Balance Challenges and Freezing of Gait

Balance changes in Parkinson's disease can increase the likelihood of falling. Reduce the risk of falls by creating a safe home environment. Place frequently used items within easy reach, remove throw rugs, place nonskid bath strips or bathmats in the bottom of the tub, and install grab bars in strategic locations near the toilet and tub or shower. Create safer habits by avoiding climbing on ladders and footstools and by sitting down to dress or shower.

Falls also increase with multitasking. Avoid carrying items in both hands and eliminate distractions when concentrating on tasks that require you to maintain balance while standing and walking.

Some people with Parkinson's experience the frustration of sudden immobility, feeling that their feet are glued to the floor. This phenomenon, known as freezing, can contribute to balance loss and falling. Compensation strategies such as imagining that you are stepping over an imaginary line or kicking through an imaginary wall of glass are often an effective means to break out of the freeze. Counting a rhythmic cadence before starting to move may also prove helpful. Marching in place with knees lifted high or rocking from side to side can help "unglue" feet and make stepping or turning easier. It is important to remain calm and avoid hurrying, which can make freezing even worse. See a physical therapist for more comprehensive evaluation of the problem and to create strategies that work best for you.

Injuries and fractures as a result of falling often lead to greater difficulty with mobility and safety. Talk to your physician about receiving a bone density test and obtaining medications for prevention and treatment of osteoporosis (decrease in bone mass and structure that makes bones weaker and more likely to break). To minimize the risk of osteoporosis, eat a balanced diet rich in calcium (found in milk, yogurt, cheese, and calcium-fortified juices and cereals). Vitamin D helps the body absorb calcium and can be made through exposure to sunlight. If you are housebound or live in a northern, cold-weather climate, a vitamin D supplement may be recommended. Weight-bearing exercises also help bones retain calcium and reduce the risk of osteoporosis.

Dizziness is a symptom that affects balance safety and contributes to falling. Some people use the term *dizziness* to describe feeling unsteady on their feet, while others report feeling as if the whole room is spinning around them. Words like lightheadedness, wooziness, or vertigo may also be used to describe this symptom. A variety of things may contribute to dizziness, including the following:

- **Low blood pressure:** Parkinson's disease and the medications frequently given for its treatment can lower one's standing blood pressure. It is recommended that individuals with Parkinson's routinely have their blood pressure monitored in both sitting and standing positions. (More on this can be found in Chapters 4 and 7 and further in this chapter.)
- **Taking multiple medications:** Taking four or more medications significantly increases the risk of side effects, including dizziness. Make sure your physician is aware of all medications you are taking and be sure to ask questions about potential side effects when starting a new prescription.
- **Inadequate fluid intake:** Dehydration can result in dizziness and loss of balance. Make sure you are drinking enough fluids, particularly during hot, humid weather or if you have been experiencing nausea, vomiting, or diarrhea.
- **Stress and anxiety:** Stress reactions can cause physical symptoms, including feelings of dizziness. Use relaxation techniques like deep breathing, soft music, or guided imagery if you are feeling stressed.
- **Use of alcohol:** Alcoholic beverages affect equilibrium and balance. Limit alcohol intake to reduce the risk of dizziness or falls.
- **Other medical conditions:** Inner ear disturbances, cardiac problems, diabetes, and depression are just a few of the many other medical conditions that may cause dizziness to occur.

Dizziness may be treated with medications, safety strategies, rehabilitation therapies, and good nutrition. It is important to report feelings of dizziness to your physician, who can make recommendations about the best options to treat your situation.

Managing Weakness and Fatigue

Some people with Parkinson's disease report feelings of muscle weakness, even when testing reveals their strength to be quite good. Slowing of motion coupled with muscle rigidity can reduce momentum and effective movement, which contributes to feelings of weakness. Some studies suggest that individuals with Parkinson's disease may have reduced core strength in the trunk and abdomen. Reduced activity and an inactive lifestyle can also contribute to loss of strength. Reports of fatigue are almost universal in people with Parkinson's disease and can combine with strength losses to further reduce activity levels. Balancing activity and rest can help reduce fatigue and enhance energy. It can be helpful to set up regular rest periods and avoid overdoing. Create an activity routine that includes stretching, strengthening, and aerobic exercises. Focus on large, exaggerated movements while exercising and throughout your daily routine because small, ineffective motions burn energy and contribute to feelings of fatigue. If tasks such as getting out of bed or rising from a chair seem difficult, separate the movement sequence into step-by-step components, focusing on each step as you perform it. A referral to physical or occupational therapy can be helpful to maximize strength and learn strategies for energy conservation.

Decide what is feasible and safe for you to perform, seeking assistance as appropriate. If feelings of weakness coincide with off periods related to wearing off of the medication, consult your physician for assistance and recommendations.

Managing Dyskinesia, Dystonia, and Wearing Off

Parkinson's medication schedules are complex, and some people notice periods of reduced effectiveness during the day or experience side effects such as dyskinesia and dystonia. It is important to take your medications on a regular schedule as prescribed by your physician. You may wish to keep a log or diary about your symptoms to share with your doctor. This can be an effective way to establish patterns of medication effects and give your physician important information for adjusting your medication schedules.

It is usually best to plan to rest and avoid strenuous activity or exercise during off periods. Use good judgment if dyskinesia affects your balance safety or driving and avoid unsafe activities. Note that attempts to stop involuntary movements by sitting on a hand, crossing the legs, or other constraints can sometimes contribute to muscle pain and discomfort. Mild stretching can sometimes help alleviate feelings of muscle cramping.

Managing Speech and Communication Problems

Loss of voice volume and imprecise speech articulation can produce communication difficulties. Reducing background noises can help eliminate competition and make your voice heard more easily. It may be helpful to sit face to face with the listener when talking. Take deep breaths and practice using your strongest voice when speaking, even if it feels too loud for normal conversation. See a speech pathologist for a thorough voice evaluation and treatment.

The saying "you can't judge a book by its cover" can easily be applied to people with Parkinson's disease. Reduced facial expression can lead to changes in communication, as most of us rely on facial expressions and gestures to interpret both the speaker's (if we are a listener) and the listener's (if we are the speaker) mood and understanding of what is being communicated. Loss of these automatic responses can be misinterpreted as disinterest, depression, or lack of understanding. Family care partners should be aware that they may need to ask direct questions about how a person with Parkinson's is feeling rather than making assumptions based on facial expressions or body postures.

Just like slowness in movement, people with Parkinson's disease can experience slowness in thought processing (**bradyphrenia**). People with Parkinson's disease may find it more difficult to respond rapidly to questions or feel that it takes longer to collect their thoughts before speaking. A quiet environment with fewer distractions is sometimes helpful in these situations. The gift of time also proves helpful in allowing the person with Parkinson's disease to express himself or herself. Family care partners may need to avoid the tendency to jump in and answer for their loved one as interruptions often make the person's thought process even more difficult.

Managing Excessive Salivation, Drooling, Oral Health, and Thick Secretions

Loss of automatic swallowing causes many people with Parkinson's to feel they have excessive saliva and occasional drooling. Sipping liquids throughout the day will ensure adequate fluid intake and promote active swallowing. Chewing gum or sucking on hard candy can also promote swallowing, but make sure the swallow mechanism works well before using these options. Avoid sugary foods, which cause increased saliva production. Some literature suggests using dried papaya, papaya juice, or even a small amount of meat tenderizer (which consists mainly of dried papaya) swabbed under the tongue to help dry excess secretions. If thick secretions persist, drinking warm broth may help. Many over-the-counter products can also help thin saliva and other secretions. Check with your doctor, nurse, or dentist.

Oral hygiene can be a challenge for people living with Parkinson's. Ask your dentist about specially shaped toothbrushes and flossing devices that may help a person with impaired manual dexterity. An electric toothbrush may also help. Scientists have confirmed that the normal bacteria that help maintain our oral health are different in people with Parkinson's disease compared to other people. Why this happens is not clear, and whether this is a cause or an effect of the changes in the consistency of the saliva that come with the disease remains to be seen. Some people with Parkinson's may choose to chew their levodopa pills. This is probably not a good idea, as the medication is acidic and can damage the dental enamel, which can facilitate the formation of cavities. Regular visits to the dentist are a must.

Severe drooling can sometimes be helped by medical interventions, including medications or injections. Consult your physician or a speech pathologist for more information on these and other options to see if they may be appropriate for you.

Managing Swallowing Problems

Approximately 50 percent of people with Parkinson's experience dysphagia (difficulty swallowing). If swallowing problems are mild, they may be helped by making appropriate menu choices, choosing foods that are soft and easy to chew. Avoid foods that are hard to swallow or have crumbly textures. Eat slowly, emphasizing a deliberate swallow or a double swallow after each bite. Alternating liquids and solids is sometimes effective. Some people use ice chips or lemon ice between bites to help facilitate swallowing. Try using applesauce or a bit of jelly to help pills slide down more easily. Avoid taking levodopa with substances containing protein, like pudding, yogurt, or ice cream, as these foods may interfere with proper absorption of the medication into your bloodstream.

If swallowing becomes more difficult or you are experiencing frequent coughing or choking, seek referral to a speech pathologist, who can provide more comprehensive evaluation and recommendations for treatment.

In the more advanced stages of Parkinson's disease, choking may become quite dangerous, even life-threatening. When foods and fluids slide down "the wrong pipe," they may end up in the lungs and cause an infection called aspiration pneumonia. In people in advanced stages of Parkinson's, aspiration may happen "silently," that is, without the patient's realizing that it happened, and lead to repeated severe pneumonia. In these cases, the doctor may discuss with the patient and his or her care partners the option of a **gastrostomy**. This is a surgical procedure that introduces a tube into the stomach through the abdominal wall so that nutrition and hydration can be provided to the individual while bypassing the mouth and esophagus, where aspiration usually happens. Some people may object to such drastic measures, and a careful conversation with the doctor is necessary. There is no universal answer as to when and whether such aggressive treatments are appropriate. The person's current quality of life, the discomforts involved or anticipated with or without the procedure, and other aspects of the person's situation must be examined in detail before a decision can be made.

Managing Vision Problems

Multiple vision problems can occur in Parkinson's disease. These include blurred vision, dry eyes, sensitivity to bright light, difficulty reading, and changes in contrast sensitivity (difficulty with vision in low-light conditions). The following are some practical strategies for coping with vision changes:

- Use artificial tears or other lubricating eyedrops regularly.
- Try using a reading magnifier or consider using large-print books or books on tape.
- Individuals with reduced vision may use contrasting colors to more easily see food on their plate, define the edge of stairs, or outline proper hand placement on a grab bar.
- Wear protective eyewear in bright light.
- Always have plenty of light to read by.

- Consult with your eye doctor about what kind of lenses to use in your eyewear. Bifocals, trifocals, and progressive lenses may increase the tendency for double vision and blurred vision in persons with Parkinson's disease.

Ask the Experts: **Managing Constipation**

Susan Imke, FNP, GNP-C, says, "Both Parkinson's disease and the medications given to treat Parkinson's can aggravate gastric (gut) problems. Maintaining good bowel function can be challenging, especially for older adults whose activity levels may be limited. The following are some suggestions:

- *"Increase water consumption to six 8-ounce glasses per day. The role of getting enough water each day in preventing constipation cannot be overemphasized. Seltzer water or club soda adds air as well as moisture to the bowel, which can increase intestinal motility.*
- *"Reduce red meat and dairy products in the diet. Limit high-fat and high-sugar foods; increase fruits and vegetables. A fruit-only snack at night and first thing each morning helps stimulate bowel action.*
- *"Increase exercise and activity levels to help keep things moving!*
- *"Drinking 6 ounces (three-quarters of a cup) of hot tea or hot water with lemon juice on arising each morning can act as a bowel stimulant. Prune juice with pulp can be helpful.*
- *"Stool softeners containing docusate sodium or an Ayurvedic combination called triphala can be used regularly. Bulking agents such as Metamucil and Citrucel provide a good fiber supplement to the diet but should not be used unless a minimum of 48 ounces of water is consumed throughout the day.*
- *"Stimulant laxatives should ideally be avoided. These products contain stronger agents, with directions to take at bedtime to produce a bowel movement in the morning.*

- *"Some patients report very good results with polyethylene glycol (brand name Miralax) taken as directed. It is now available over the counter, but its use should be approved by your doctor or nurse practitioner.*
- *"If these measures are not enough to prevent or manage chronic constipation, your physician can recommend prescription medications to use for a limited time.*
- *"Try not to sit on the toilet for longer than 5 minutes or strain to pass hard stool. The goal is to honor the body's natural urges over attempting to produce a bowel movement on schedule."*

Managing Difficulties with Bladder Control

Bladder changes in Parkinson's can include **frequency** (needing to urinate often), **urgency** (feeling as if one needs to urinate immediately), or difficulty with fully emptying the bladder. These bladder difficulties sometimes prevent people with Parkinson's disease from drinking enough fluids because they try to avoid a sudden need to use the bathroom. Remember to drink fluids throughout the day, even if not feeling thirsty. Some people find it helpful to limit their fluid intake in the evening hours to prevent frequent nighttime trips to the bathroom. Individuals with both bladder urgency and mobility problems may wish to consider obtaining a urinal or bedside commode for nighttime use.

Another reason that some people have to get up in the night to use the bathroom is that they have ankle swelling. All the fluid that accumulates in the feet and ankles throughout the day reenters the circulation once the person is reclining, and the kidneys try to rid the body of the extra fluid by producing more urine. If this is a problem, medications to reduce swelling, the use of elastic stockings, or simply elevating the legs in the evening a few hours before bedtime may reduce the nocturnal frequency.

Speak with your physician about any bladder problems you are experiencing. Sometimes a specific physical therapy called pelvic floor exercise or medications can be helpful (see also Chapter 7). Developing a regular schedule for toileting may also help with bladder control. Choosing clothing that is easy to remove in the bathroom (e.g., garments with elastic waistbands and without complex fasteners or belts), use of incontinence pads, or both may help reduce stress and frustration about getting to the bathroom promptly.

Dealing with Loss of Mobility in the Advanced Stages

Individuals living with advanced-stage Parkinson's may experience significant limitations in mobility. It is important to maintain a regular schedule for changing positions throughout the day and night to maintain adequate circulation and skin integrity. Try to change position at least every hour during the waking day and every 2–3 hours at night. A caregiver may need to assist with these position changes. The use of pillows or cushions can help one maintain a comfortable position and good body alignment. Rubbing skin with lotion or oil can also help circulation and prevent redness or pressure areas.

If mobility changes make regular walking difficult, a wheelchair may be needed for transport around the home or community. Make sure the wheelchair is fitted properly for the user's height and body size and obtain a cushion for the seat, back, or both to maintain proper positioning in the chair.

Dealing with Mild Cognitive Symptoms

Some people with Parkinson's disease experience changes in concentration, memory, or processing of information. These changes, although not always severe, can be frustrating in daily life. A calm environment free of distractions can help a person with such difficulties focus attention on the task at hand. Multitasking and multiple-step processes (e.g., following a recipe) can be especially challenging for persons living with Parkinson's disease. It is important to create an environment that will allow concentration on the task at hand. Distractions while driving can have dire consequences for anyone, but particularly so for people with Parkinson's.

Keep eyeglasses, keys, and other regularly used items in consistent assigned places to prevent hunting for lost or misplaced items. Countless people with Parkinson's disease have fallen and injured themselves while frantically looking for their keys, coat, and other items when running late for an appointment. Many people find it helpful to keep a calendar of appointments and events as a memory aid for their scheduled activities. Practicing trivia, crossword puzzles, sudoku, or other "neurobics" games can help keep your thinking skills sharp.

Managing Confusion, Hallucinations, and Dementia

If thinking changes become more severe, it is important to take steps to ensure the individual's safety and comfort. To prevent confusion, caregivers can help create an environment free of clutter or unneeded items. Remove medications or small items that could be mistaken as food items from places the person with Parkinson's can reach. Installing safety latches on basement doors or cupboards containing hazardous products can help prevent accidents.

It is not usually advisable to argue with someone who has dementia or hallucinations, as it can result in escalating confusion or agitation. Try to maintain a calm environment, keeping your voice volume low. It can sometimes help to distract the person by changing the subject, offering a rest period, providing a snack, or suggesting an alternative activity. Care partners should plan for increased confusion or even agitation with any change in their loved one's environment, such as taking a trip, staying at an unfamiliar place, or moving into a new living environment.

Rapid changes in thinking can be the result of illness, infection, or injury. Bladder infections, which may occur without any alarming symptoms, are notorious for causing sudden changes in the mental function of people with Parkinson's and dementia. Some medications can also cause confusion or hallucinations as a side effect. Caregivers should consult the patient's physician if they observe sudden thinking changes.

Dealing with Apathy, Depression, Impulsivity, and Anxiety

Many symptoms related to Parkinson's involve a person's emotional world. Changes in mood and personality can occur. Some patients develop apathy: the loss of interest, motivation, and initiative. This may result in a decreased desire to participate in activities the person enjoyed in the past or a tendency to sit passively for extended periods. Encourage the person to exercise and engage in other activity throughout the day. Even short periods of movement help to improve circulation, reduce muscle stiffness, and maintain motor function. A care partner often must take the initiative. Patients with Parkinson's who experience apathy will still enjoy their favorite activities once someone else gets them going.

Depression is often seen in Parkinson's and is related to the chemical imbalance in the brain. It is important to address feelings of depression or note changes in sleep patterns, appetite, or mood with your physician. Many people with Parkinson's benefit from prescribed antidepressant medications. Others find counseling, exercise, support groups, or other activities to be helpful in coping with depression. A combination of many strategies is usually the most effective management. Care partners need to be on the alert for signs of depression in the person with Parkinson's. Any suicidal thoughts should trigger an immediate call to the person's physician or to a crisis-consulting agency. Be aware that the risk of suicide may be somewhat higher for the first few weeks of treatment with certain antidepressants as well as after DBS surgery. Such times require increased vigilance on the part of the care partner.

Impulsive behaviors (trying to move too quickly or engaging in unsafe behaviors such as climbing and overreaching) are sometimes seen in patients with Parkinson's disease. Impulse-control disorders (compulsive gambling, eating, or shopping; hypersexuality) have been linked to the use of some dopamine agonist medications. Make sure to discuss any impulsive or compulsive behaviors with your physician, even if the activity does not seem harmful (e.g., cleaning or rearranging furniture). Medication adjustments may be warranted.

It is estimated that approximately 40 percent of people with Parkinson's experience anxiety. This can range from a mild anxiety disorder to panic attacks and is sometimes linked to the person's medication schedules or wearing off. Medications and counseling can be helpful in managing anxiety. Other activities, such as deep breathing, biofeedback, meditation, tai chi, and yoga, are sometimes helpful. Make sure to report any feelings of anxiety to your treating physician or healthcare provider for recommendations most suitable to your situation.

Managing Sleep Changes in Parkinson's Disease

Many factors contribute a restful night's sleep. Parkinson's disease can interrupt the sleep cycle at both ends of the spectrum, creating insomnia for some people and drowsiness for others. Medication side effects can worsen sleep changes by causing excessive sleepiness or frightening nightmares. Practical strategies to help ensure good rest include the following:

- Try to stay on a regular schedule, keeping bedtime consistent.
- Get adequate exercise.

- Avoid excessive daytime sleeping.
- Limit fluid intake after 7 PM if bladder changes result in frequent nighttime trips to the bathroom.
- Use satin-based nightwear or a slippery fabric drawsheet in the middle third of the bed to make rolling and getting up from bed easier.
- Use a lightweight comforter to avoid having multiple sheets and blankets, which can get tangled up with your feet and restrict bed mobility.
- Keep the bedroom at a comfortable temperature for sleeping.
- Seek a referral to physical or occupational therapy for advice on safe and comfortable positioning and techniques for getting in and out of bed more easily.
- Contact your physician for advice on medication adjustments if immobility prevents you from rolling in bed or getting into bed safely at night.
- Report feelings of restless legs, frequent nightmares, or "acting out" dreams to your physician.

Managing Orthostatic Hypotension

Orthostatic hypotension—low blood pressure made worse by rising from a chair or bed—can occur in people with Parkinson's disease. This can lead to feelings of dizziness, vision changes, difficulty thinking clearly, or fainting. Falls can also occur. The following actions can help deal with orthostatic hypotension:

- Have your blood pressure checked in both seated and standing positions.
- Avoid rapid position changes. Sit on the edge of the bed before getting up. Stand for a moment after rising from a chair to make sure you are not feeling dizzy.

- Maintain adequate fluid intake. Dehydration can cause even larger drops in standing blood pressure.
- Consider when dizziness or fainting episodes occur. Many people notice increased difficulty immediately after eating a full meal, when their digestive system requires increased blood flow. If these episodes are worse after meals, consider eating smaller, more frequent meals during the day.
- After being seated for longer periods, move your arms and legs around to stimulate circulation before getting up.
- Seek advice from your physician, nurse, or dietitian about increasing your salt intake, which may help keep blood pressure from dropping.
- Wearing elastic support stockings is sometimes helpful, but they may be difficult to put on and wear regularly. Abdominal binders or compression undergarments are sometimes recommended. Ask your medical team members for their input and recommendations.
- Some people benefit from the use of medications to keep standing blood pressure at higher levels.

Weight Loss

Medication effects, difficulty swallowing, depression, and other medical factors can contribute to weight loss in people with Parkinson's. If unexpected or unwanted weight loss occurs, include calorie-dense foods at mealtime and eat between-meal snacks, drink liquid supplements, or both. Remember that slowed movements can affect chewing and swallowing and may cause someone to fatigue before finishing a meal. Parkinson's disease causes the stomach to move—and therefore empty—more slowly, which can cause a feeling of fullness early in the meal, a condition called early satiety. Try smaller, more frequent meals if fatigue or early satiety becomes an issue. Seek a referral to occupational therapy if you are having difficulty with the mechanics of eating, such as managing silverware and cutting food. Vision changes in contrast sensitivity may make it more difficult to see food on the plate. Use color-contrasting dishes when possible to compensate for these visual changes. Your physician, nurse, or dietitian can provide additional recommendations. Swallowing difficulties should be assessed by a licensed speech pathologist. In the end stages of the disease, maintaining proper nutrition may require the placement of a gastrostomy tube (see Managing Swallowing Problems previously presented in this chapter). If weight loss occurs despite adequate nutrient intake, it's very important to consult with your general practitioner or internist to look for other possible causes.

Keeping Skin in Shape

People with Parkinson's may experience increased redness, flakiness, or irritation of their skin. This is called seborrheic dermatitis, and it is more prominent around the nose, eyebrows, and forehead. Although it is rarely a serious problem, the following tips will help keep seborrheic dermatitis under control:

- Wash affected areas daily using a mild, bland soap (Basis, Dove, or Ivory). Rub gently.
- Apply 1 percent hydrocortisone cream (available over the counter at drugstores) sparingly to affected areas.
- Mild astringents such as witch hazel can be used to reduce oiliness.
- Control dandruff or flaky scalp with shampoos that contain selenium (Tegrin, Neutrogena T/Gel).

People with Parkinson's disease have an increased risk for melanoma (a dangerous form of skin cancer). Check your skin regularly for any changes. Avoid too much sun, particularly between 10 AM and 2 PM and in midsummer. Sunlamps and tanning beds should also be avoided. Use a sunscreen with a sun protection factor (SPF) of fifteen or higher, even on cloudy days. Apply the sunscreen thoroughly to all exposed skin, including around the eyes, ears, and mouth and on any areas on your head that are bald or have thinning hair. Ultraviolet (UV) rays can penetrate through loosely woven clothing, so wear sunscreen even on areas covered by clothes. Apply non–oil-based moisturizing lotion after a bath or shower. A lip balm with the sunscreen para-aminobenzoic acid (PABA) and UV-opaque sunglasses are also recommended.

Hospitalization

Health changes or injury may result in a hospital stay. Parkinson's disease symptoms may escalate during periods of illness or injury, so many people require more assistance than usual for general mobility. Hospital medications are often given on set schedules different from what the person with Parkinson's disease is used to, compromising mobility further. Bed rest may increase feelings of stiffness and muscle rigidity. Hospital staff may not be familiar with Parkinson's or the unique needs of the patient with Parkinson's.

Make sure you carry a detailed list of your medication schedule with you, and work with the hospital to receive your medications according to this timetable. Ask your attending physician to write specific orders about the importance of medication timing. Even after doing these things, difficulties may still occur, as hospital schedules are not usually set up to accommodate special requests or timetables. A family care partner may need to advocate for a person with Parkinson's disease who is ill or injured. Some hospital settings will allow the patient or care partner to assume responsibility for administering Parkinson's disease medications.

Health professionals unfamiliar with Parkinson's may not fully understand motor fluctuations or changes in a person's ability to walk, eat, or dress through the course of the day. Reinforce with the hospital staff the concept that some people with Parkinson's disease move differently at certain times of the day, and let the staff know that you may need more assistance during off periods. Do not hesitate to ask your attending physician to consult with your neurologist, who may be able to give additional information about your overall health history as well as provide useful advice about things such as needed medication changes or drugs that should be avoided.

Try to get up and start moving as soon as possible during the hospital stay, but always with your treating physician's consent. Seek a referral to physical therapy to provide bedside exercise assistance if you are unable to get up and ask to begin a course of rehabilitation therapies before discharge to restore flexibility, strength, and endurance. For more prolonged hospitalizations, a period of inpatient rehabilitation at a specialized facility may be necessary.

The Parkinson's Foundation has created an Aware in Care kit designed to help individuals with Parkinson's and their families advocate for receiving Parkinson's pills on time while in the hospital. This free kit can be obtained by contacting the Parkinson's Foundation (see Appendix).

Elective Surgery

In deciding whether to undergo elective surgery (e.g., joint replacement and cosmetic procedures), it is important to carefully consider the potential impact of Parkinson's disease. Seek input from your neurologist or movement disorder specialist to discuss your plans and receive appropriate recommendations.

Most surgeries will cause an interruption in your medication schedule. Make sure the surgeon is aware that you have Parkinson's disease and will need your medications resumed as soon as possible following surgery. Some surgical procedures may allow you to take your Parkinson's disease medications with a sip of water even on the morning of surgery, but you must receive clearance from the surgeon before doing so. Some Parkinson's medications may not mix well with certain anesthetics, and your surgeon may ask you to stop them weeks in advance. In such instances, always check if that is safe to do with your neurologist, as some of these medications should not be discontinued abruptly. There is a long list of medications that people with Parkinson's disease should not take because they may make their symptoms worse. Unfortunately, with the standardization of procedures at hospitals, orders for such medications may be entered automatically. Therefore, always be aware, to the best of your ability, what medicines you are given and for what reason. For example, many nausea medications and tranquilizers should be avoided in people with Parkinson's.

As your body undergoes the stress of recovery, be aware that it often takes longer for people with Parkinson's disease to resume a normal routine after surgery. Follow-up rehabilitation therapies can help restore function, whether provided at home, in a transitional care setting, or on an outpatient basis. It is important to remain as active as possible within recommended restriction guidelines. Don't forget the importance of good nutrition and adequate rest throughout the recovery process.

Medications to Avoid

Medications that block the action of dopamine should not be given to people with Parkinson's disease unless they have been shown not to worsen the symptoms of the disease or unless they are absolutely necessary. Such medications are called antidopaminergic drugs and are used mainly to treat nausea, slow stomach movement, and psychotic symptoms such as hallucinations and paranoia. Some common antipsychotics are haloperidol (Haldol), chlorpromazine (Thorazine), and risperidone (Risperdal). Metoclopramide (Reglan) is an antidopaminergic medication often used for stomach trouble. Many antinausea medications, such as prochlorperazine (Compazine), trimethobenzamide (Tigan), and promethazine (Phenergan) work through blocking dopamine actions and can worsen the symptoms of Parkinson's disease; promethazine is also used as an antihistamine. Always check with your doctor and your pharmacist to determine whether it's OK to take any newly prescribed drug with your Parkinson's.

CHAPTER 10

Lifestyle Changes and Disease Management

In this chapter, you will learn about

- Lifestyle changes that will improve your life with Parkinson's and long-term outlook, such as exercise and the therapeutic value of music and dance
- Leisure time, driving, and travel
- Stress management, spirituality, and community involvement
- Complementary therapies and medical cannabis

The Importance of Exercise

Michael is an active 44-year-old man who has been living with Parkinson's disease for 4 years. He loves to run for exercise and fun. Since his diagnosis, he has continued to run about 2 miles a day, performing regular warm-up stretching before hitting the streets. Sometimes, Michael experiences dystonia (painful muscle cramping and abnormal foot posturing) while running. As a result, he's adjusted his schedule to exercise at times he feels his medication is working best.

Susan is a 57-year-old woman who has been living with Parkinson's for 3 years. She works full time as a billing clerk at a local hospital. Because she's tired after work, Susan has adjusted her schedule so she can go for a 30-minute walk before heading to the office. She also uses a yoga DVD at home several times a week and feels that regular stretching provides her with the greatest benefit in reducing her feelings of muscle stiffness. At work, she performs brief stretches she learned in physical therapy to combat neck and shoulder stiffness.

Paul is a 70-year-old man who was diagnosed with Parkinson's 7 years ago. Although retired, he maintains an active lifestyle and enjoys travel, gardening, and golf. Paul attends a local health club 3 or 4 days per week, where he uses the strength-training machines, treadmill, and stationary bike. Paul gets advice from a personal trainer at the club. He finds this keeps him motivated to exercise.

Irene is an 82-year-old woman who has been living with Parkinson's disease for 15 years. She recently completed physical therapy and is following through with a home exercise program designed to work on her flexibility, leg strength, balance, and walking skills. Irene spends approximately an hour each day working on these activities, focusing on making large, exaggerated motions while exercising. Her husband provides her with support and assistance as needed. Irene has also begun to participate in an exercise group at a local Parkinson's center twice a week.

Exercise is an important component of an integrated treatment plan for Parkinson's disease. Although the individuals described are all quite different, they have all taken steps to incorporate exercise into their daily routine. The benefits of exercise are many, including improved strength, bone health, flexibility, and endurance. Recent studies suggest that exercise may have a disease-modifying effect on Parkinson's by helping remaining dopamine cells to function more efficiently. Researchers from the Parkinson's Outcomes Project found that people with Parkinson's who engage in at least 2.5 hours of exercise a week had better quality of life than those who didn't exercise at all. Research has also suggested that for people with Parkinson's to receive maximal benefits, exercise must challenge the individual by being specific, intense, and repetitive. (See more on exercise in Chapter 7.)

Many types of exercise programs are appropriate for patients with Parkinson's disease. Some people enjoy tai chi or biking, while others prefer treadmill training, walking, or yoga. You may have heard about

Parkinson's-specific programs, such as LSVT-BIG, Parkinson Wellness Recovery, Rock Steady Boxing, and Delay the Disease. No one specific program or protocol is right for all people with Parkinson's. It is most important to choose a safe program that you enjoy and will be motivated to continue on an ongoing basis. A physical therapist can help you design a program that works well for you, and it will be helpful to check in with your therapist and update your program on a periodic basis.

Here are several tips to consider with respect to exercising with Parkinson's disease:

- Take your general health into account when planning your exercise program. Consider any condition or past injury that could be aggravated by increased activity and check with your physician and physical therapist regarding the appropriateness of your planned program.
- Set realistic goals, creating an exercise program that fits into your schedule and budget. Setting a regular time for exercise each day will help you adhere to your routine. Every person is different, but it is often helpful to choose a time to exercise when you are usually functioning well and are not too tired.
- Make sure you include activities that promote flexibility, strength, balance, and cardiovascular conditioning in your routine. Exercises promoting trunk flexibility are very important, even in early stages of the disease. Exercises designed to improve core strength (abdominal and trunk muscles) are also recommended. Consider programs such as tai chi or yoga, which offer an integrated approach that promotes stretching, strengthening, and balance training. In addition to the usual exercise benefits, a walking program gives you an opportunity to improve your walking pattern by focusing on large steps and wide turns while walking.
- If balance changes make standing or walking exercises unsafe, design your program so that you do most exercises while

lying down or sitting. Maintaining a good general activity level is also important. Gardening, yard work, golf, tennis, and household chores all contribute to the overall value of exercise, but they cannot substitute for a structured exercise program.

- Contact a physical therapist or an exercise physiologist for an evaluation and assistance in developing an appropriate exercise program. Membership in a local health club may offer access to equipment and skilled staff who can provide guidance. Joining a community exercise class or group sponsored by a health facility or senior center can also help you stick with the program through the support and encouragement of other class participants.

Ask the Experts: I Have Been Diagnosed with Parkinson's. What Should I Watch or Change in My Diet?

Susan Imke, FNP, GNP-C, says, "A frequent question asked by those living with Parkinson's disease is 'Should I be following a special diet?' In general, people are encouraged to eat a balanced diet, with foods from all four basic food groups (fruits and vegetables, grains, meats, and dairy). A healthy diet usually limits red meat and avoids foods high in salt, processed sugar, and saturated fats. Many dietitians recommend augmenting a well-balanced diet with daily vitamin and mineral supplements as a nutritional 'insurance policy,' taking these supplements with food. It is not advised to choose a megadose vitamin formula.

"There is growing evidence that foods rich in antioxidants may have health benefits for everyone, including people with Parkinson's disease. Many antioxidant supplements purchased without a prescription do not affect brain health, because they are unable to cross the protective blood-brain barrier. Natural antioxidants found in foods are able to enter the brain and are

most plentiful in foods such as fruits and vegetables, walnuts, green tea, grape juice, red wine, and dark chocolate.

"Medications used to treat the symptoms of Parkinson's disease may be affected by when and what types of food are eaten. Proteins found in food compete with levodopa for absorption in the stomach and small intestine. So it's best to take levodopa on an empty stomach. Four or five ounces of nondairy fluid taken with the levodopa tablet before eating (even 15 minutes before may be enough) will propel the drug faster through the stomach and into the small intestine, where it will get absorbed into the bloodstream. Think of it as giving the levodopa a head start on absorption over the food about to be eaten.

"Typically, the people most affected by protein are those who experience significant on/off motor fluctuations, those who take levodopa four or more times per day, or both. To verify if protein is interfering with levodopa absorption, experiment with a vegetarian diet or move the daily recommended allotment of protein to the evening meal. Altering the timing of protein intake may help prevent interference with levodopa absorption. Reducing overall amounts of daily protein may also prove helpful, but note that protein is important to overall nutrition and that even those people who are 'protein sensitive' should not try to eliminate protein from their diet. It is advisable to avoid taking levodopa-containing medications with milk, yogurt, pudding, or other protein-rich foods. Consult with your physician to see if other dietary changes are advisable. Referral to a nurse or a licensed dietitian familiar with Parkinson's disease for additional recommendations may also be helpful.

"Nausea can occur as a side effect of medications. If levodopa causes nausea, a small cracker or bite of fruit can be taken with doses required between meals. Pretzels are excellent, because they require no refrigeration. Crystallized ginger can be nibbled to offset nausea.

"Parkinson's disease may affect the ability to eat and digest food efficiently. Just as it causes slowness in movement, Parkinson's also slows gastric (gut) motility. In patients with Parkinson's, chewing and swallowing may be prolonged, stomach emptying may be delayed, and food moves through the intestines more slowly relative to someone who does not have the disease. For all these reasons, nutrients may be better absorbed when the person with Parkinson's eats small amounts frequently rather than three large meals per day.

"As eating and digestive processes slow down, weight loss can become a problem for many people who have Parkinson's. Frequent, small meals can help them to maintain optimal weight. Liquid supplements can be useful. Sometimes patients are so diligent in limiting fat intake and worrying about protein restrictions that they deprive themselves of much-needed calories.

"Maintaining adequate fluid intake may become more difficult for people who have difficulty swallowing or who are reluctant to drink liquids because of the bladder changes sometimes seen in Parkinson's. Our natural sense of thirst may diminish with age, and anti-Parkinson's drugs also dry out the body. It is important to drink water 'by the clock,' not unlike the way one schedules crucial medications. This allows better absorption of nutrients from foods as well as of medications and reduces the risk of dehydration."

Leisure Activities

Generally, it is important to stay active when living with Parkinson's. Recreational activities provide physical, mental, and social stimulation and keep us connected with friends and family. Keep your physician and other team members informed if you have experienced significant changes in your pursuit of leisure interests because of mobility challenges, depression, or anxiety.

Many people with Parkinson's report that they feel at their best when engaged in activities they truly enjoy. Hobbies and leisure interests promote relaxation and are essential to replenish mind, body, and spirit. It is wise to make a commitment to ensure adequate time for leisure pursuits within your regular schedule. Although Parkinson's disease can change involvement in past interests, simple adaptations may allow continued enjoyment of leisure activities. For example, avid gardeners may wish to consider installing raised flower beds to improve access to their garden space, and cyclists may want to try using a recumbent bike to continue riding.

Remember that Parkinson's often makes movement slower and can affect balance. To ensure safety, proceed cautiously when attempting activities you have not performed in some time. Remember that warm-up stretches help prepare stiff and rigid muscles for activity. Be mindful that fatigue or off time also affects your ability to fully engage in more active leisure pursuits. Remember to take medications with you and keep taking pills on schedule.

Changes caused by the disease also create opportunities to try new leisure interests. Exploring new activities promotes creative expression and enhances quality of life. Many people have been pleasantly surprised to discover a hidden talent for creative outlets such as painting, writing, sculpting, or photography that was unrecognized before their diagnosis of Parkinson's disease.

Stress Management

We live in a world of schedules, deadlines, and multitasking that often increase stress levels. Most people with Parkinson's find that physical and emotional stressors often make their symptoms worse. When under emotional stress or when fighting a cold or flu, they may experience increased tremor, slowness, or other symptoms. Some patients note increased difficulty with Parkinson's symptoms if they feel worried, anxious, or upset. To help reduce stress, here are strategies some people with Parkinson's disease are using:

- **Judy, age 62:** "Placing all my appointments and commitments on one calendar reduces chances of overbooking my schedule. I schedule my rest breaks, too!"
- **Michelle, age 57:** "I have revised my wardrobe to get rid of blouses with small buttons, jewelry with small clasps, and other items to make my morning routine flow more smoothly."
- **Jose, age 68:** "I take just a few minutes to do some stretches for my neck and shoulders each morning. I find it much easier to put on my coat, a task that used to make me very frustrated each time I prepared to leave the house!"
- **Gary, age 47:** "I give myself extra time to get out the door for work, church services, or scheduled appointments to reduce feeling hurried or rushed."
- **Sadie, age 72:** "I have finally learned to say no. It's a simple word but often difficult to say. Agreeing to too many commitments builds stress in my daily life."

Some people with Parkinson's find it helpful to schedule time for relaxation each day. Simple deep-breathing exercises can reduce stress and promote relaxation. Use of soft music or relaxation tapes can also prove helpful. Massage, active exercise, and meditation are also used by many to combat stress levels.

People living with Parkinson's disease often experience anxiety disorders. Significant feelings of unmanageable stress, anxiety, or panic should be discussed with a physician. He or she can assess the need for treatment with medications and make referrals to a social service agency or a mental health professional. (More information on anxiety can be found in Chapters 4, 7, and 9.)

Driving

Depending on where you live, the ability to drive may be an important part of daily life. Slowed movements, vision changes, neck stiffness, and difficulty with multitasking caused by Parkinson's disease can all have a negative impact on safe driving. Here are tips to make driving easier:

- Alter your driving schedule to avoid peak traffic and times when your medications are not working well.
- Reduce night driving if Parkinson's is affecting your vision in low-light settings. A 2009 study published in *Neurology* found that, compared with the general population, patients with Parkinson's have double the risk of automobile accidents when driving in fog or low light.
- Because people with Parkinson's can have difficulty with multitasking, focus your attention on the road by turning off the radio, not talking on your cell phone, and avoiding other distractions.
- Get out of the car frequently to stretch and move around. Remember to stretch your neck and shoulder muscles, too.
- Make sure your car seat offers good support or obtain a support cushion for improved posture and driving comfort.

The time may come when the ability to drive safely becomes too compromised by Parkinson's symptoms. Each person must maintain honest self-assessment or obtain feedback from trusted friends or family members on whether it's still safe to drive. For more formalized assessment, seek a referral to an occupational therapist who can perform a driving evaluation and offer recommendations for changes or modifications.

Ask the Experts: I Have Been Diagnosed with Parkinson's Disease; Should I Stop Driving, and, If Not, What Should I Be Watching For?

Ergun Y. Uc, MD, has the following advice:

- *The diagnosis of Parkinson's disease in itself does not automatically disqualify you from driving.*
- *Parkinson's disease is a long-lasting illness, and many patients continue driving after the diagnosis.*
- *The decision whether to continue driving depends on how the disease affects specific functions such as vision, attention, information processing, decision-making, multitasking, memory, and reaction speed.*
- *Fitness to drive in Parkinson's disease decreases over time; however, Parkinson's affects every individual differently.*
- *Periodical evaluation by different experts (e.g., neurologist, primary care doctor, neuropsychologist, occupational therapist, physical therapist) along with input from the family and friends may be needed to reach a decision that balances independence of the patient and safety.*
- *As long as patients with Parkinson's disease are deemed safe to drive, they should heed the following to reduce risk of crashes:*
  - *Only drive while your medications are working and you are not tired.*
  - *Be familiar with the car you are driving.*
  - *Do not drive in inclement weather with poor visibility and slippery roads.*
  - *Plan your driving routes ahead of time.*
  - *Avoid congested traffic, unfamiliar surroundings, and left turns at busy intersections.*
  - *Avoid multitasking, such as using your phone, eating, or engaging in heated conversations.*

> - *If your medications wear off or you feel tired/sleepy, take a break.*
> - *Always carry your cell phone with you for emergencies.*
> - *Develop alternative transportation plans for poor driving conditions and plan ahead for the future to reduce dependence on driving.*

It is wise to plan ahead and consider alternative transportation for when driving independently is no longer an option. Carpools or public transportation may be options for some people. Others may need to make arrangements for rides from friends, neighbors, and family members. Some communities have volunteers who will drive patients to medical appointments, grocery shopping, and other errands. In addition, many religious entities (e.g., churches, synagogues, and mosques) help arrange rides to attend religious services.

Using Complementary Therapies

Many people with Parkinson's disease choose to explore the use of complementary or alternative therapies. While evidence-based research in this area that indicates clear benefits is still lacking, many people try acupuncture, massage, and a variety of other complementary options for overall health and wellness. One study suggested that less than one-half of people with Parkinson's who use complementary therapies report them to their physician. A survey of 435 people with Parkinson's found that almost two-thirds had tried at least one kind of complementary therapy, such as massage, yoga, tai chi, meditation, or acupuncture. Most people with Parkinson's who tried these therapies found them effective. Most people (85 percent) who tried meditation found it very helpful, and most of the people who participated in the survey indicated a strong interest in further exploration of complementary therapies. It is always preferable to openly discuss all treatments you are using with your healthcare providers to ensure they have a full understanding of all aspects of your health.

Cannabis

It would be an omission not to touch on the subject of medical cannabis, as much information is available on the Internet and not all of it is reliable. This is a rapidly changing field, and we can only recommend caution. Cannabis is often touted as "nature's miracle." The use of cannabis to treat neurologic diseases is grounded on the fact that the human brain contains specific proteins called receptors that are responsive to cannabinoids, a class of compounds found in cannabis. These receptors may act as a switch that activates and deactivates certain nerve cells in the brain and thus may alter certain brain functions. Different types of these receptors have been found in the human brain, and scientists have determined that one type of cannabinoid receptor, labeled CB1, is less abundant in the brain of people with Parkinson's. Researchers have conducted some small trials with cannabis in Parkinson's and found that in certain cases, it may alleviate tremors and dyskinesia. However, the authors of these studies have cautioned that there is still too little information about how to properly use cannabis in Parkinson's, whether more purified components should be evaluated separately, and, more than anything else, how safe it is to use such products in people with Parkinson's, who may often be of older age and may have other health problems. The safety of long-term use of cannabis is still a matter of scientific debate, even when it comes to the young and healthy brains of college students, and we have to ask the question of how safe it will be when used in people who are older and have a disease that is attacking their nervous system.

Regarding the more practical aspects of medical cannabis, its use is legal in some, but not all, US states, and different countries have different laws covering its use. Although medical use of cannabis may be allowed in certain states, its use may be restricted to specific diseases, and Parkinson's may not be one of them. Where the use of recreational marijuana is allowed, caution is needed, as the available products may not have a similar content of active ingredients and may lead to adverse side effects. A person with Parkinson's and early dementia may develop severe hallucinations and end up in the hospital if he or she uses a cannabis product that contains higher levels of tetrahydrocannabinol (THC), which is one of the active ingredients in cannabis, or a product that may have been laced with stronger opioids. Over-the-counter cannabis-derived products are also available and used to calm anxiety. Be aware that some surveys of preparations available in the market have shown inconsistencies in content of the various ingredients; therefore, if you plan to use these products, it is wise to discuss first with your Parkinson's specialist or nurse.

> **Cannabis products** may help tremors, dyskinesia, and anxiety in Parkinson's disease; however, they should be used cautiously and after a discussion with a healthcare provider.

Spirituality

Living well with Parkinson's requires attention to mind, body, and spirit. The diagnosis of Parkinson's affects plans and dreams for the future. This altered path can contribute to feelings of bewilderment, anger, and sadness. It is important to acknowledge these feelings and grieve the associated losses. Many people turn to their spiritual beliefs to help make sense of their feelings and emotions. It is normal to ask "Why me?" or to seek a higher power to help deal with this unforeseen event. Sorting out your emotions by exploring your beliefs and values is a normal process toward building resiliency and hope.

Hope helps us live with unpredictability and see our situation in a new light. Most organized religions and spiritual beliefs are built on a foundation of hope. Even people with advanced symptoms of Parkinson's disease single out feelings of hope as a powerful tool in coping with the challenges of everyday life. Some studies have cited a connection between prayer and health outcomes.

Not all people view spirituality as being connected with organized religion. A connection to nature, keeping a journal, meditation, and use of inner resources such as optimism, humor, and motivation can all be manifestations of spirituality and may be powerful supports for those living with Parkinson's disease.

Travel

Whether it is related to business or pleasure or is frequent or rare, it is likely that people with Parkinson's will want to travel. However, travel plans may need to be changed to accommodate challenges caused by Parkinson's. It is advisable to choose your itinerary wisely. Ask questions before you start. It's important to conduct research on the area to which you will be traveling, accessibility issues, and time schedules for the trip. Itineraries that provide flexibility, luggage assistance, and easy-to-negotiate surroundings may be best. If necessary, find a travel agent who is willing to work with you to design an ideal travel experience. If you want to have grab bars, accessible showers, and raised toilet seats available, make an advance request for accessible hotel accommodations or cruise cabins. Schedule time for rest as needed. Take an extra day on arrival or before departure to rest before you set out on your travels or arrange to stop along the way for a refreshing break.

Make sure your luggage is lightweight and has wheels. When flying, remember to keep medications in carry-on luggage, not in a checked suitcase. It is advisable to carry extra medication with you in case of travel delays. Minimize your luggage, but make sure you take items that are necessary for a good travel experience. If you sometimes use a cane or walker, take it with you. This advice is sometimes ignored but shouldn't be. So, we'll say it again: if you sometimes use a cane or walker, take it with you.

Change position frequently when traveling. When driving long distances, stop every hour or so for a brief stretch. When flying, perform shoulder shrugs, ankle circles, and neck and arm motions.

If flying, you may wish to request an aisle or bulkhead seat to allow for extra legroom. To decrease travel stress, use skycaps, airport wheelchair assistance, and luggage porters. If possible, avoid checking wheelchairs or walkers. If traveling with a wheelchair, walker, or cane, keep it with you until you arrive at the flight gate for boarding and request that it be returned to you as soon as you get off the plane. Take advantage of calls for preboarding to give yourself extra time. If your medications need to be given by injection (e.g., apomorphine), you may need a note from your doctor to be allowed to carry the necessary supplies on board with you.

Being outside your normal living environment can sometimes prove disruptive. Consider any time changes within your itinerary to adjust your medication schedule accordingly. You may need to improvise if you normally use adaptive equipment to make daily life easier. For example, a straight-backed chair against the side of the bed can serve as a makeshift bed rail.

It is wise to ask for advice and help when needed. Hotel concierges, cruise pursers' desks, and Chamber of Commerce travel information stops can provide information and assistance for persons with physical mobility challenges. Above all, try to have fun! Travel can be an adventure, even if it is common to experience delays and disruptions in routine.

The Power of Music and Dance

Music and rhythm have been shown to have an impact on the nervous system. We are all aware that certain types of music raise our spirits and make us want to move, while others help us relax and unwind at the end of a long day. Research in music therapy for Parkinson's has demonstrated that moving to music can help an individual achieve better range of motion, improve walking cadence, and reduce freezing. Use of a metronome or music with a steady beat provides a backdrop to help set the pace and keep people with Parkinson's moving more easily.

Music also evokes beneficial emotional responses. Creative musical activities such as improvisation, drumming, songwriting, and discussion of lyrics have been used successfully to help individuals express their thoughts and emotions, reduce stress, and find a sense of accomplishment.

Several studies have recently been published indicating the benefits of dance in people with Parkinson's disease. Individuals participating in dance classes twice a week showed improvements in balance, functional mobility, and walking. Active exercise combined with the benefits of enhanced movement through music and rhythm is the suggested basis for such improvements.

Music therapists are trained professionals who offer therapeutic interventions to restore, maintain, or improve function using music. Neurologic music therapy is a type of music therapy specialized for treating neurologic patients. Neurologic music therapists work in a variety of care settings, although they may not be as common as other therapists on an interdisciplinary team. In many states, music therapy is not eligible for insurance reimbursement. To find a music therapist in your area, visit the American Music Therapy Association website at *musictherapy.org*.

Getting Involved in the Parkinson's Community

Meeting other people with Parkinson's and sharing common concerns in a support group setting can be very helpful. A number of online and in-person support groups are available. Some groups are geared more for the recently diagnosed or those with young-onset Parkinson's. It is usually best to do some initial investigation so that you can find out more about a group's goals, its format, and who usually attends before deciding if it will be a good fit for you. Joan was diagnosed with Parkinson's disease 10 years ago and helps to facilitate the local support group in her community. She considers her support group members part of her team and knows that they help her to stay positive. "I may also help others when sharing what works for me!"

There are also opportunities for involvement in Parkinson's research studies. These can take the form of surveys, medication trials, interviews, or other types of participation. It is important to ask questions regarding the study's design and any potential benefits or risks before deciding to participate. Your physician may be aware of research studies in your area, or you can investigate a number of ongoing studies online.

Some people with Parkinson's disease choose to become involved through advocacy, fundraising, or volunteerism. Many people feel that a sense of involvement in such activities contributes to overall quality of life. Contact a local or national Parkinson's center or organization to learn more.

Although there are a variety of ways to become involved in Parkinson's-related activities, each individual must decide her or his own level of interest and comfort in doing so. Some people find it upsetting to be involved in activities with other people with Parkinson's who may be in a more advanced stage of the disease. Some are not comfortable sharing their thoughts and feelings in a group setting. Mel has Parkinson's disease but clearly states that he does not consider himself a "group person." Rather than joining a support group, he found meaning in joining his local Parkinson's boxing class and becoming involved in the community speakers' bureau of the local Parkinson's organization. "These things reinforce that I am not alone and allow me to focus on what's right instead of what's wrong. Parkinson's is a significant part of my life, but it is not my whole life." There is no right or wrong decision on getting involved; the decision is yours. (Chapter 13 has more information on community involvement and advocacy.)

Ask the Experts: How Should I Prepare for Doctors' Appointments?

Susan Imke, FNP, GNP-C, has the following advice:

- *"Choose your healthcare providers carefully. You should feel confident in their knowledge and understanding of Parkinson's disease. You should feel comfortable asking questions. You should feel like your concerns are being addressed. If possible, seek care in a Parkinson's specialty clinic.*
- *"Try to arrive for scheduled appointments a few minutes early, giving yourself adequate time to complete the check-in process and any paperwork.*
- *"Bring a current list of medications to all medical appointments. Include the medication names, dosages, and timing schedules. This is particularly important in a new care setting or an emergency department.*
- *"Bring someone with you to neurology appointments to share observations that supplement your own report and to listen carefully to the advice or directions you are given.*
- *"Think about priorities for your appointment beforehand and jot down questions so you'll remember to ask them. If your list is long, be aware that you may not be able to discuss every issue and may need to make a follow-up appointment.*
- *"Be your own best advocate! Your physician is a capable coach of your healthcare team, but you are the owner. Familiarize yourself with the role of all team members, such as rehabilitation therapists, social workers, and nurses. Seek referrals to other professionals as questions or problems arise.*
- *"Make sure you understand all instructions before leaving your appointment. Ask questions if instructions are unclear.*

- *"Provide necessary information to ensure that reports are sent to your other physicians and healthcare team members. Sign the necessary medical release forms and have complete names, addresses, and phone numbers of these healthcare team members readily accessible.*
- *"Keep telephone reports brief and to the point; when possible, speak for yourself.*
- *"If you need to be admitted to a hospital, transitional care setting, or nursing home, be aware that many of the staff are unlikely to have special expertise in Parkinson's disease. Your medication schedules are likely to be disrupted. Be prepared to provide information or answer the same questions repeatedly. Caregivers may need to step in to advocate for someone with a recent illness or injury."*

More on choosing your doctor and the roles of the members of your healthcare team can be found in Chapter 5.

CHAPTER 11

Research

In this chapter, you will learn about

- Reasons that people choose to participate in Parkinson's research

For most people living with Parkinson's disease, research represents the hope of a cure, and this hope is what often triggers a desire to participate in experimental trials. Before deciding to become a volunteer for Parkinson's disease research, it is important to learn about the types of research studies that may be available. It is equally important to understand one's own reasons for agreeing to participate in research and realize that there may be risks, both evident and hidden, associated with such decisions. In this chapter, we provide some basic information about research to answer some of the most frequent questions and concerns that surround decisions on whether to take part in research.

Why Should I Consider Participating in Research?

People with chronic illnesses are often drawn to research because they hope that research will give them a chance to receive newer, better treatments or maybe even a cure. Although hope is a good thing, this is probably the wrong reason to become a volunteer for research. The word *volunteer* here is used intentionally; becoming a research participant or a research subject, as studies often refer to participants, is an act of volunteering. The best reason for participating in research is a desire to help science progress toward better treatments and eventually a cure. Without volunteers, research cannot progress, and 10 or 20 years from now treatments for Parkinson's will not be any more effective than they are today. Only one thing can change this, and that's research.

At the center of the research effort stand the many people with Parkinson's disease who volunteer to become subjects. Although volunteering may sound too altruistic, participating in research does often provide some "fringe benefits." For one, it gives a person with Parkinson's disease the opportunity to fight back. The research volunteer becomes a soldier in an army fighting for the cure. Just as in a war, battles may be won or lost, but what motivates the fight is the hope for the final victory, even though it may take years to get there. Besides this feel-good benefit, participating in research usually involves receiving very detailed evaluations and tests, which may discover and result in the treatment of other, unsuspected health problems.

> Volunteering **to participate in research helps improve our understanding and treatment of Parkinson's.**

Albert was in his late 40s and had just been diagnosed with Parkinson's disease when he agreed to participate in a placebo-controlled (this term is explained further in this chapter) research trial of a new medication that had shown promise for slowing the progression of the disease. As part of the screening tests, he had to see a dermatologist (skin specialist) for an examination.

The dermatologist had bad news and good news for Albert. She pointed out a small dark spot on Albert's back, which he and his family physician had never noticed before. She told Albert that this was likely a melanoma, a form of skin cancer that can be life threatening if not treated in the early stages. The dermatologist removed the lesion, which, indeed, turned out to be a melanoma, and reassured Albert that the cancer had been detected and treated early enough to not be a cause of concern anymore. Albert was unable to be part of the research study, but his decision to volunteer to do so may have saved his life.

What Kinds of Research Studies May Be Open to a Person with Parkinson's Disease?

You may be able to participate in two types of research studies. The first type does not involve investigating a form of treatment. Studies of this sort are usually **observational**, and their aim is to better understand the symptoms of Parkinson's disease, the development and evolution of such symptoms over time, and the risk factors leading to such symptoms. Observational studies also investigate the possible causes (genetic or environmental) of the disease. The second type of study is called interventional. Such studies evaluate the potential benefit of an "intervention," whether a new drug, therapy, or surgery.

Observational Studies

Here are some examples of observational studies:

- A scientist (in this case, an epidemiologist) wishes to find out if caffeine consumption decreases the risk for Parkinson's. He may design a questionnaire to determine how much caffeine a person has consumed in the past 5 years. He will then administer this questionnaire to two groups of people, one group with Parkinson's and one group without, and compare the results.

- Another scientist may want to take this question a step further and study whether caffeine consumption has any impact on how fast the disease progresses. This scientist may ask people living with Parkinson's to record all the forms of caffeine they consume over, for example, 5 years. After 5 years, the data can be studied to determine whether the rate of progression correlates with the amount of caffeine consumed.

Similar observational studies may investigate how genetics, family history, amount and type of exercise, lifestyle, other health problems, or even socioeconomic factors may influence the risk of developing Parkinson's disease, the rate at which the disease progresses, or the types of symptoms a person develops once he or she gets the disease. The goal of such research, besides trying to predict how some patients may fare compared with others, is to generate ideas about what kinds of changes a person can make to improve her or his own outlook. Such ideas can be further tested with interventional studies (see the next section). One such example would be that if an observational study shows that people with Parkinson's who exercise regularly do better over the years than those who don't, one could design an interventional study to see if asking patients to exercise alters the course and prognosis of the disease.

Interventional Studies

This second type of research in which people with Parkinson's disease may participate examines the effects of specific treatments (interventions) on Parkinson's disease. The treatment under study may be a new and promising medication, a new type of surgery, a nutritional supplement, or a type of therapy or exercise. The scientists who design such a study specify a hypothesis they want to test. An example of a hypothesis is that Drug A improves the motor symptoms of Parkinson's disease. The scientists also specify the ways that improvement will be measured. In the same example, they may decide that the effectiveness of the drug will be measured by comparing patients' scores on the Unified Parkinson's Disease Rating Scale (UPDRS; see Chapter 2) before and after treatment with Drug A. They may go as far as specifying, for example, that they expect at least a 10 percent improvement and, based on that expectation, do some statistical calculations to figure out how many people should participate in the study. (As a rule, a study needs more participants to detect a smaller effect.)

One important aspect of such studies is the **placebo**. It is very well known that when a new treatment is tried, both the patients who receive it and the doctors who administer it may see improvement in the symptoms even when the new medication is not truly effective. This can even happen when patients are given a pill that contains no medication whatsoever. The word *placebo* refers to such a sham treatment, and the improvement seen with ineffective medications or placebo is called the placebo effect. The placebo effect is a sort of wishful thinking, and it can be very strong; in fact, it has been shown to be fairly strong in Parkinson's disease. It is not clear why the placebo effect happens, but it probably has to do with the power of suggestion and the hope created by the simple fact that one is trying something new and promising. Unfortunately, the placebo effect is short-lived and without any long-term benefits. Therefore, sham pills are not really useful to treat any diseases.

Because of the placebo effect, most well-designed interventional studies come with two important qualifiers: placebo-controlled and double-blind. Placebo-controlled means that a portion of the participants will receive a sham intervention, be that a "sugar pill" (it's actually usually a flour pill) or a noneffective form of treatment. For studies of surgical treatments, some participants may actually receive a sham operation! Then, the improvement in the group of participants who received the treatment under investigation will be compared to the improvement, if any, in the placebo group. The second qualifier in these studies, double blind, means that neither the participants nor the doctors who assess the results of the treatment under study know who receives that treatment and who receives the placebo. This way the doctors can be objective in their assessments, and the wishful thinking effect is minimized.

Interventional studies assess not only the effectiveness but also the safety of new treatments. Many of these treatments, particularly medications, have not been used widely, so the full range of their potential unwanted side effects may not be well known. Therefore, a risk may be attached to participating in such studies. For this reason, participants in drug trials usually undergo very extensive medical testing, such as repeated blood tests, electrocardiograms, and urine analysis. Some studies may involve more sophisticated testing, like positron emission tomographic (PET) scanning, magnetic resonance imaging (MRI), or a lumbar puncture (also known as a spinal tap). With some studies, participants may be asked to provide a sample for analysis of their genes (DNA analysis).

In the United States, drug trials of new medications are supervised by the FDA with a very rigorous process to maximize safety and minimize mishaps. Any serious reaction to the medication during the trial must be immediately reported to the drug company that produces the medication and to all the doctors participating in the study. External monitoring committees review all the test results to ensure that no patterns of serious complications emerge as the study progresses. Finally, the physicians who conduct the study are supervised by the institutional review boards (often referred to as the IRBs) of their own institutions. Such multiple levels of supervision and double-checking help ensure not only the validity of the study results but also the well-being of the participants.

Informed Consent

Because of all the concerns mentioned in the previous paragraphs, people who agree to participate in research must read and sign an "informed consent" document. This document contains a lot of information about what the study entails, how many visits are required, what kinds of tests will be performed, what potential side effects are already known, and what types of side effects might be possible based on the available scientific knowledge about the particular treatment. For example, an experimental drug may not be known to cause liver damage; however, based on its chemistry, scientists may have reason to believe that it has the potential to cause such damage. In that case, frequent testing of liver function may be required by the study design (usually referred to as the study protocol).

It is very important to carefully review the informed consent and have all your questions answered to your satisfaction before signing it. Your signature means that you agree (that is, consent) to participate and that you understand the potential risks and effort involved (that is, you are informed). However, your signature is not a contract, which means that it does not legally bind you in any way. You retain the right to withdraw your consent to participate at any point throughout the study. You will also be given contact information for people you may notify if you suspect that the study is not conducted properly. Conversely, the study physician may withdraw you from the study if she or he believes that continuing the study may be detrimental to your health or if your further participation may compromise the scientific integrity of the results (e.g., if something happened that convinced your doctor that the diagnosis of Parkinson's was wrong in your case).

Clinical drug studies are classified as phase 1, 2, 3, or 4 studies. These are the phases of testing the drug in humans after it has already been extensively tested in experimental animals. Phase 1 studies test the safety of the drug and find out the necessary and safe dosage in healthy volunteers and persons with the disease of interest—in this case, Parkinson's. Phase 2 studies focus on drug safety in a small number of persons with Parkinson's while also assessing the drug's effectiveness. Phase 3 studies examine long-term effectiveness and safety in larger groups of patients with Parkinson's. Phase 2 and phase 3 studies usually have strict inclusion and exclusion criteria, so people who may have many other health problems or are on too many medications may be excluded. Phase 4 studies are usually "open label" (which means no placebo is used) and are done after the drug has gained approval by the FDA to better assess how it performs in the real world. Phase 4 studies are very important because they can assess the usefulness and safety of the new drug among the kinds of patients who were excluded in phases 2 and 3.

Where Can I Learn More?

Whether the research study in which you wish to participate is observational or interventional, make sure you understand all the details before you make up your mind to participate. Inquire about your alternatives and always ask about the risks and effort involved. You may get more information about clinical trials in Parkinson's disease from your healthcare provider, local academic institutions, the organizations listed in Appendix A, and the following sources:

- National Institutes of Health: *clinicaltrials.gov/*
- US Food and Drug Administration: *fda.gov/science-research*
- Michael J. Fox Foundation: *foxtrialfinder.michaeljfox.org*
- Parkinson's Foundation: *parkinson.org/research*
- American Parkinson Disease Association: *apdaparkinson.org/ research*

CHAPTER 12

The Care Partner

In this chapter, you learn about

- Being a care partner for a person with Parkinson's
- Resources for care partners
- Planning for the future
- How others have dealt with Parkinson's affecting a loved one

Many people do not like being called a "caregiver." That's because they may not provide hands-on care, or they don't like a label that suggests some degree of disconnection from their loved one. Some prefer the term *care partner*, recognizing that coping with Parkinson's disease requires a true partnership. We use these terms interchangeably throughout this chapter, but we prefer care partner. No matter what term is used, it is important to acknowledge that both lives affected by the diagnosis, after which things are never quite the same. Once someone is diagnosed with Parkinson's, a new era has begun for both that person and his or her spouse, partner, or significant other.

Even though a care partner may have recognized changes in the loved one for some time, the official diagnosis of Parkinson's often comes as a shock. A common reaction is feeling overwhelmed. How can the doctor know for sure? Shouldn't tests be done? Should we get a second opinion? (In many cases, that's a good idea.) As medical evaluations and care proceed, it's often helpful for care partners to accompany their loved ones to appointments to learn about Parkinson's disease.

Care partners are also involved in seeking out information and doing initial research into the diagnosis. Seeking appropriate educational literature through credible organizations and websites can be helpful, although it may be best not to bombard your loved one with every detail you learn about Parkinson's disease. Care partners may be even more overwhelmed than patients with the implications of a chronic neurologic condition. An informed care partner can be helpful to the loved one by providing reassurance that Parkinson's disease is highly "livable," progresses slowly in most patients, and does not appreciably shorten life expectancy.

Discuss together how you will share the news of the diagnosis with friends and family members. If you have children living at home, choose a level of information and an approach that is age appropriate. Learning about or visiting a support group is helpful for some people, but it is important to do your homework and find a group that's a good match for your situation. Recently diagnosed people (and their care partners) may be overwhelmed by support groups made up primarily of individuals who have lived with Parkinson's for a long time. What's more, a recently diagnosed person's concerns will probably not be addressed in the most appropriate manner in such a group.

Be prepared for an initial onslaught of free advice. Friends and adult children are notorious for suggesting miracle cures they've heard about, herbal supplements, or the latest article they've just read online about Parkinson's disease. Patients should talk to their physicians before proceeding with any of their recommendations.

The care partner will need to recognize that Parkinson's disease causes slowness of movement and feelings of fatigue. Patience and a good sense of when help is needed are often required from the care partner. Avoid the tendency to do everything for the person with the disease. Most people prefer to be independent and may resent attempts to provide assistance. Care partners are often helpful simply by being flexible, recognizing that Parkinson's disease symptoms may result in changed schedules and plans. Knowing that stress exacerbates symptoms can help care partners understand that asking someone to hurry usually makes the situation even worse.

Worry or concern over a loved one's diagnosis of Parkinson's disease is normal. In the early stages of Parkinson's, the daily routine may not be disrupted. It is often not necessary to make major life changes. If changes or accommodations become necessary, it is important to recognize that care partners still need to fulfill their own needs to maintain their health and wellness. Try to keep connections with relatives and friends who nurture your spirit and continue to make time to do things you enjoy.

The rate of symptom progression in Parkinson's disease varies considerably from one person to another. Care partners are urged not to predict problems but to be prepared for changes that are likely to occur over time. As time goes by and symptoms increase, care partners often need to make additional adjustments. In time, fluctuations in the response to levodopa (e.g., wearing off, on/off phenomena, and dyskinesia) may appear. These fluctuations make it hard to plan activities or predict physical capabilities, since Tuesday may be different from Wednesday. Recognize that these fluctuations are part of Parkinson's disease for many people and are not under your loved one's control. It is important to try to be flexible when scheduling activities and events. At the same time, it's important to realize that loss of motivation and even depression can be part of the disease. Sometimes the care partner must be the motivator, and it may be challenging to balance encouragement to do more things and keep active with backing off and letting your loved one rest.

People with Parkinson's and their care partners rarely adjust to living with the disease at the same rate. Role conflicts often emerge at this stage of the illness. Renegotiate who can and will do which tasks. (Who should pay the bills? Is it time to hire someone to do the yard work? Is continued driving by the person with Parkinson's beginning to affect the safety of family or others on the road?) These conversations can be difficult because they reflect the patient with

Parkinson's enormous loss of independence and may result in more responsibility and stress for the care partner. As Parkinson's disease progresses, changes in mood and cognition (how the person feels, thinks, and reasons) may become more problematic than motor symptoms. Seek medical guidance when noticing increasing physical symptoms (e.g., slowness, walking changes, or balance loss) or mental changes affecting safety (e.g., confusion, hallucinations, paranoia, or dementia). These changes can sometimes be improved with medication adjustment, but they may also signal needs for further adjustment in the daily routine.

Coping with Caregiver Stress and Fatigue

Realistically, caregiver stress is just part of life when caring for a loved one over an extended period. The term *caregiver burnout* is sometimes used in the literature but suggests the unfortunate image of a flame extinguished with no hope of relighting the wick. Caregiver distress can be acknowledged and managed only if the person in distress or close, caring observers take notice of the warning signs and are willing to intervene.

Early signs of caregiver fatigue may include the feeling that after several years of increasingly taking the lead in your relationship (with no end in sight), life is not turning out the way you'd expected. Voice your concerns and seek assistance as needed. Don't attempt to become a superhero. Maintain open communication with your loved one and allow time and opportunity to candidly discuss your fears and concerns. Midstage Parkinson's disease may also prove an ideal time to share more details about the disease with key friends and family members. If you haven't done so already, make sure crucial planning documents, such as a **will**, a durable **power of attorney**, and advance directives, are in place (more on this in Chapter 14). Start building your backup team, people who can help you out in small ways now and familiarize themselves in ways to help if they need to fill in for you in the future when the need becomes greater.

Signals of increasing caregiver fatigue can take many forms. Fatigue may include growing feelings of isolation. The feeling that "nobody knows or understands what is really going on with us" is always frustrating and is sometimes true. The care partner may have increasing feelings of anxiety or uncertainty about the future, and his or her patience may be tested, resulting in outbursts of anger, often followed by feelings of guilt. Stressed care partners often report feelings of profound tiredness or exhaustion not relieved by sleep. Stress-induced physical symptoms (e.g., recurrent headache, upset stomach, and other pain) may also occur. Some caregivers develop problems concentrating and making decisions. They can experience feelings of depression, bitterness, despair, and hopelessness. These warning signals are not to be overlooked. Caregivers should seek medical evaluation for any physical symptoms and discuss any feelings of stress or depression with a medical provider. Many care partners benefit from counseling, antidepressants, support from social services, or other interventions designed to help them cope with increasing fatigue.

Caregivers may wish to acknowledge their stress levels and fatigue by scheduling a meeting with key friends and family members to candidly discuss what's happening in their lives. Have the courage to share feelings of isolation, disappointment that friends have stopped coming to visit, or frustration that family members are not supportive in the ways you need. Make a short list of specific tasks that would help you take better care of your loved one and get some much-needed respite. For example, a caregiver could ask a friend, "Could you come on Tuesdays to take Frank to the barber or out to lunch?" Be honest if lack of funds is a constant worry; perhaps someone in your circle can help with medication costs for 1 month or pick up groceries for you once a week. Ask for one or two volunteers to be "on call" for you during particularly bad days.

If symptoms reach advanced stages and the person with Parkinson's requires even more care and support, it often becomes difficult to separate yourself from your role as a caregiver. It is vital to establish a pattern of taking care of your own physical and mental health needs as well as those of the person with Parkinson's. Don't put off scheduling a mammogram or neglect a morning walk because you feel too busy or preoccupied meeting a loved one's needs. Martyrdom is overrated as a coping mechanism! (If you failed to establish yourself as a priority early on, it's never too late to start.)

Private time and relaxation are basic human needs. Make an effort to schedule time away from caregiving responsibilities on a regular basis. Consider drafting a written caregiving plan that specifies that you get, for example, 1 hour per day and 1 day per week to yourself. To continue giving effectively to the other person, it is essential for long-term caregivers to restore their own energy and recharge their batteries on a regular basis. This may even involve something as simple as turning off the cell phone and checking into a nearby hotel. Call on the people who have prepared and trained to serve as your backup team. This is not selfish. If you become ill or suffer severe burnout, who would possibly be there in the same way for your loved one?

Accept assistance when it is offered but be mindful of potential caregiver burnout even in your local helpers. For instance, an adult daughter living nearby with a job and children at home may feel as overwhelmed as you do. Be frank with long-distance family members regarding how they might help. For example, suggest they come and fill in for that long weekend, pay for dental work not covered by insurance, or cover the prescription copay that's become out of financial reach. Family members and friends can also help by phoning every week at an expected time or just sending a card every month; such small gestures can provide amazing comfort amid great distress.

Home care services can assist with caregiving tasks such as bathing and dressing and with other personal needs. If you can afford it, consider paying someone to clean the house and perform household maintenance. Some home care services are covered by insurance, but many require adequate private funds for payment. A social worker or geriatric case manager can help you access available home care services in your community and offer guidance regarding fees and services provided.

What Can I Do to Keep Up with the Demands of Being a Care Partner?

One care partner compared her experiences to running a marathon. It's "long and sustained, sometimes tiring, at times feeling never-ending, although ultimately a gratifying experience." Both care partners and marathoners need to follow some of the same basic rules to be successful:

- Train and prepare. Take time to learn about Parkinson's disease and what to expect if symptoms progress. Seek a care partner support group or other venue where you can share your thoughts and feelings with others with similar experiences. Ask questions during medical appointments and seek referrals to social services, counseling, and other support as needed.
- Replenish energy along the route. While time away is important for needed respite, don't underestimate the power of even a short break in the daily routine. A brief walk, a phone conversation with a friend, or just a cup of tea and a favorite TV program can help restore perspective and energy.
- Protect the body to avoid injury. Make sure you receive proper instruction in how to best help your loved one. Learn about use of good body mechanics and techniques to safely help your loved one out of chair or off the floor after a fall or to transport a walker or wheelchair in your car. Seek referral to a physical therapist who can instruct you in these matters and so reduce the risk of your being injured.

- Rest before and after "the race." Schedule breaks into your day and make sure you are getting enough sleep. Consider arranging overnight assistance a few times each week if you are not receiving adequate rest. Use of the services of adult day programs or volunteer respite programs may allow you time for daytime sleep.
- Sometimes walk part of the way. No one can do it all, including family caregivers. Recognize that despite your best efforts, some days do not go as planned. Consider ways to simplify the daily routine and try to reduce any tendency for perfectionism. Keep a few frozen dinners stashed for emergency use, learn to say no to outside requests from others, or make use of delivery services to cut down your daily to-do list.

Planning for the Future

Be proactive as you consider future plans. These questions are worth discussing with family members and others:

- What will we do if my loved one becomes ill and requires greater levels of care?
- What will we do if I become ill or am no longer able to provide care to my loved one?
- What will we do if neither of us is able to remain in our current situation?

If you are concerned about needing a different place to live for you, your loved one, or both of you, investigate in advance the need for and availability of assisted-living and skilled nursing facilities. It may also be helpful to familiarize yourself with palliative (comfort) care options and hospice programs, so if and when the need arises, you will know where to turn.

Take a friend, relative, or geriatric care manager with you to visit a few places and get an idea of the available choices. This is easier than waiting until a hospital stay and discharge necessitates finding a place on short notice. A list of appropriate questions when reviewing senior residential communities or nursing homes may include the following:

- Has the staff received training/education to better understand the needs of those with Parkinson's disease?
- What is the look and feel of the facility as you walk in? Would you be proud for friends and relatives to visit you here?
- How far is the available unit from the dining area? Is everything on one level?
- Are there appealing views or outside spaces?
- Do things seem clean and in good repair?
- Is there a laundry facility for residents?
- What is the level of noise and chaos in the common areas?
- Does the facility have specific memory care/dementia areas or programs?
- Are you comfortable talking with the marketing director and other staff you meet? How long has the chief administrator held that job? Is a registered nurse available or on call 24/7?
- Do you feel pressure to "decide today" and sign move-in commitment forms? Is there an option to "try before you buy" by staying in a guest room and taking multiple meals in the facility to see if it is a good match for your needs and preferences?
- What do residents say about the food service and dining room staff? Are serving hours flexible? Can the cook accommodate special requests, such as eggs cooked to order? If you are unable to come to the dining room, what is the charge for a tray brought to your room?
- In addition to the basic monthly charge, how much are fees for services such as help with bathing and dressing and medication

assistance? Who determines what services you need? Can additional services be added to your monthly bill without your prior permission?

- Are hairstyling services available on premises? What is the cost for a haircut, style, or manicure?
- What days are transportation services available? Is help available for getting into and out of the van and handling packages? Do these services cover the area where your doctors' offices are?
- In the event of a medical emergency, can you be taken to the hospital of your choice?
- Does the facility have rooms available for people on Medicaid-funded programs, so that you can remain there if your personal funds are spent? What percentage of residents pay out of their own pocket?

If you are a care partner who is an adult child, friend, or other relative, you may consider moving the person with Parkinson's disease into your home. Be realistic and consider all options. Ongoing caregiving can bring out the best and the worst of many situations. Your freedom to come and go on short notice may be sacrificed, and caregiving may take time and attention away from other family members, who may act out in unanticipated ways. While children in your home may need to be quieter as a result of having an older relative in the home, older children and teens may become kinder, more thoughtful family members. You may be surprised to find out that friends or other family members can become critical or offer unwelcome advice once you have taken in the person with Parkinson's disease. Although the person you care for may be grateful for your help, be prepared for times he or she appears unpleasant or resentful of the need for constant care. Despite the burden of caregiving, the relationship between you and your care recipient can become stronger over time.

A Care Partner's Story: Marilyn

Although she's married, 73-year-old Marilyn does pretty much everything around the house these days. "I cut the grass, grocery shop, cook, clean, wash, iron, shovel the snow, take the dog to the vet, take him [her husband, Jim] to the doctor, pick up all the prescriptions, and make the dental appointments," she says. "Sometimes," Marilyn adds, "I feel like I'm being pulled in a hundred different directions."

Marilyn's husband was diagnosed with Parkinson's 10 years ago. Jim is in his mid-70s now. The disease wasn't bad at first; he had a tremor on one side of his body and had trouble remembering the plots of movies. But over the years, things have slowly become more difficult for Jim—and Marilyn. When he gets dressed, he often misses a button on his shirt or a belt loop on his pants. Because of tremor, he also has trouble combing the back of his hair and shaving his face. He can do it—it's just that he misses spots. When his nose drips, he doesn't notice. So Marilyn has to help him, remind him, prod him.

"I feel more and more overwhelmed," she says. "I'm overwhelmed physically, financially, and emotionally."

Lots of caregivers feel like Marilyn. Taking care of a loved one while taking care of yourself and a house is a big, big job. It's also a job that requires more time than most paid jobs. Here are some of the strategies Marilyn uses to cope. They can be useful strategies for all caregivers to consider

- Attending support group meetings. Marilyn attends a caregivers' group that meets every other Monday at a local senior center. The other group members provide tips and share stories. "Listening to the stories helps me know what to look for in the future," Marilyn says. "It's been a great help."
- Exercising regularly. In the summer, Marilyn works in the flower garden, tending to her hostas and ferns. Because gardening reduces the stress in her life, Marilyn calls the flower

garden her "stress garden." In the winter, she walks on the treadmill in her living room.

- Making time for friends. Jim is well enough to go fishing with his buddies and—with the help of family—to be on his own occasionally. So Marilyn schedules regular breakfasts and lunches with friends from high school. Since they've known each other for more than 5 decades, she feels like she can tell them anything.

- Making necessary changes in the house. Marilyn and Jim love each other, but they sleep in twin beds now because Jim gets up frequently in the middle of the night to go to the bathroom. The noise wakes up Marilyn, but the twin beds allow her to get a good night's sleep. They've also added a railing to Jim's bed to make it easier for him to get out of bed.

- Asking for help when she needs it. Marilyn's adult children live nearby, so sometimes she asks for help with big outdoor chores. They've got busy lives, but somehow, they find the time to lend a hand. Although she takes pride in doing all the housework herself, she hired window washers for the first time in more than 50 years because she just can't do everything.

- Planning for the future. Marilyn and Jim have their wills and power of attorney documents completed (see Chapter 14).

- Not doing everything. Jim needs lots of help, but he's not helpless. Once when he asked Marilyn to look up a phone number for him, she encouraged him to find it himself. Although he ultimately couldn't find it without help, she felt the nudge encouraged him to be independent in areas where he is capable.

- Enjoying the little things. At about the time Jim was diagnosed with Parkinson's disease, the couple bought a miniature schnauzer. The dog has been a great companion for Jim, following him around the house and joining him on the recliner at night. And when Jim goes to bed, the dog curls up with Marilyn.

A Care Partner's Story: Rich

"Parkinson's is a disease that you must take a day at a time and respond to whatever challenges that particular day brings. An extra phone call or trip to the doctor may not provide any relief, because the problem of the day may simply be the general progression of the disease. On the other hand, since the disease causes changes in the patient, a conversation with the doctor may result in a modification in medication or a change in some recommended therapy that may help return the quality of life closer to normal.

"As each day brings its own challenges, there is nothing better for the patient than to know his family and caregivers are ready, willing, and able to help in any way that is necessary. Our family always tried to be there for my father and to help with his special requests when my mother was not able to do so. We always encouraged him to get out of the house and even simply run errands with my mother just to give him a change of scenery and get his mind off the constant worry about the progression of the disease."

CHAPTER 13

Community Involvement, Advocacy, and Resources

In this chapter, you will learn about

- Ways to become involved in the Parkinson's community
- How others with Parkinson's have tried and succeeded in making a difference
- Some resources for community involvement

Parkinson's disease isn't just about medication, coping, and loss. Many people find that becoming active in a support group or advocacy organization adds a sense of belonging and purpose to their life. That is also true for people with Parkinson's disease, their care partners, and families.

Attending support group meetings to share common problems and worries is helpful for many people. A number of support groups are available, both online and in person. Some groups focus on the recently diagnosed, care partners, or people with young-onset Parkinson's disease. Before attending a meeting, it's a good idea to find out more about a group's audience and goals to see if it's a good fit for you.

Opportunities for involvement in Parkinson's research studies are also available. These studies come in a variety of forms, such as surveys, medication trials, or interviews. It is important to ask questions about the study's design and any potential benefits or risks before deciding to participate. Your physician may be aware of research studies in your area, or you can investigate a number of ongoing studies on your own. (Chapter 11 has more information on research.)

Although there are a variety of ways to become involved in Parkinson's-related activities, each individual must decide on his or her own level of interest and comfort in doing so. Some people find it upsetting to be involved in activities with other people who are in more advanced stages of the disease. Some are not comfortable sharing their thoughts and feelings in a group setting. There is no right or wrong decision on getting involved. The decision is yours.

Some people with Parkinson's disease choose to become involved through advocacy, fundraising, or volunteerism and feel that a sense of involvement contributes to their overall quality of life. To find out more, see the Appendix for a list of associations and organizations for advocacy opportunities. In addition, many US states are home to local affiliates of these national organizations. Visit their websites or call the organizations for information on local chapters and events.

A Passion for Advocacy

Jackie Hunt Christensen has always been a bit wonky. After college, she worked as a public policy advocate for Greenpeace and then shifted her emphasis to agricultural trade issues. "I've always worked for action-oriented organizations," she says. "It's a natural thing for me."

At age 32, Jackie suspected something wasn't quite right with her physically. Two years later, she was diagnosed with Parkinson's disease. She soon became a fierce advocate for people living with the disease. She served on the board of directors of the Parkinson Association of Minnesota (now a chapter of the Parkinson's Foundation), coordinated state efforts for the Parkinson's Action Network, and even organized a 1-day Parkinson's conference at a local university.

"It's in my blood," she says. "I feel like if I'm not doing something actively to make life better, the disease wins. I'm not ready to concede that yet."

Jackie has also written two books: *The First Year: Parkinson's Disease: An Essential Guide for the Newly Diagnosed* and *Life with a Battery-Operated Brain: A Patient's Guide to Deep Brain Stimulation Surgery for Parkinson's Disease*. Not everybody has to be as involved as Jackie to have an impact on the lives of others. In fact, Jackie wishes lots of people would take small steps to help the public better understand Parkinson's disease.

"In my definition of advocacy, anyone who doesn't let the disease keep them imprisoned in their own home is an advocate," she says. "Simply by going outside or going to church and being willing to answer questions, you are an advocate." Jackie believes that people need to be educated about an issue before you can get them to do something. So, educating someone in your neighborhood; a member of your church, synagogue, or mosque; or anyone else about the disease makes you an advocate. Most people have an extremely limited view of what Parkinson's disease is. By asking questions, they are showing a desire to learn more. Jackie hopes more people living with Parkinson's will help educate folks.

"I feel strongly that the actual patient voice needs to be adequately represented," she says. Jackie recommends first talking to others one on one about the disease and then becoming comfortable talking to small groups at a place of worship or local civic organization.

"Ease into it," she says. As for Jackie, she's also going to keep advocating for people with the disease and their families.

"I can't imagine not being able to do this."

A Passion for the Arts and Helping Others

Bright colors illuminate the paintings of Sheila Moriarty. Sometimes the colors are magnificent, as in the sweeps of orange, green, and yellow that fill a rendering of flowers. In other works, the colors are subtle. In one painting of a church on a winter day, the eye is drawn to snow clinging to a barren tree. But soon it drifts to a bluish green sky that suggests a wish for spring.

Sheila didn't begin painting until she received a diagnosis of Parkinson's disease. She paints with watercolors because it's less time-consuming than other forms of painting.

"I only work in watercolors because it's fast," she says. "I fear I don't have much time before my medication wears off." She adds, "I paint for the love of it."

But Sheila's not the only one who loves the paintings. Her paintings have been purchased at art fairs, church sales, and silent auctions. The Parkinson's Foundation has featured her watercolors on its website, and a Scottish Parkinson's organization has adopted one of her paintings as its logo. Sheila also often donates paintings to fundraisers for Parkinson's-related causes because she wants to make a difference in the lives of people. "It gives me a thrill, because it's like I'm part of the research team," she says. "I can help."

Sheila isn't the only one who feels this way. Many people with Parkinson's disease or family members of someone with the disease feel empowered by giving back to the community. They do it in lots of ways.

Mike Justak is an individual with Parkinson's with a need to educate and inform others. His unique project is an annual holiday light show in sync to music called PD Shimmers. Mike's idea is to raise awareness of Parkinson's disease by shining one light for each person diagnosed with Parkinson's each year. That amounts to a neighborhood home display of over 58,000 lights organized and set up by volunteers! Those who come to view the display learn facts about Parkinson's through the synchronized radio station that plays the holiday light show music. Attendees are also invited to make a donation to the Parkinson's community. "It's been my lifeline. It's been a passion, without a doubt. It's a way to remind people that there are 1 million people with Parkinson's in the United States," Justak says.

When Parkinson's made it more difficult for him to organize the show, his whole neighborhood came to help.

Of course, there are plenty of more conventional ways to raise money for Parkinson's advocacy and research. Many state organizations sponsor walkathons, bike rides, golf tournaments, bowlathons, charity runs, tea parties, auctions, bake sales, and other community events.

Some Final Thoughts

Annie offered some final thoughts on living with Parkinson's:

"When the future appears dark, I remind myself it could always be darker. If I wake up in a bad mood or have difficult symptoms, I go for a walk with my dog. Sometimes I can't get my legs to cooperate with walking, and dog and I simply have to stay close to home. But we still walk. Sometimes we "sit-walk." We feel the breeze, hear the sounds, smell the smells (dog does, anyway), and enjoy the sun.

"Another important aspect of staying positive is to do something that helps someone else. It can be something as simple as writing a hello card to a friend, neighbor, or relative. I also allow myself to do something nice for myself; I get a massage, indulge in a good book, or have lunch with a friend.

"Parkinson's is not going to go away for me, although I do have hope for new treatments that eventually will stop the progression or cure the disease. For now, I savor every moment, laugh at silly things, cry when I'm sad, and mostly just appreciate the world around me. I know it isn't simple to put things back together after a setback, but even tiny baby steps move us toward a better mind-set.

"Parkinson's changes the lives of all the people it touches: the person living with it, the caregiver, siblings, children and grandchildren, friends, and neighbors. I remember my former self

and I wish I wasn't changing. I feel bad for myself, but I feel worse for my spouse and kids. I wish they didn't have to do so much for me. I wish I didn't get worn out so easily and fall asleep on the couch. I wish a ski vacation included me on skis. I wish I could show them that I know how to play shortstop. I wish they didn't need to hold me up—both literally and figuratively. I am in awe of their compassion, resilience, optimism, patience, and love.

"I know that Parkinson's is a sneaky, opportunistic disease. It introduces itself with small annoyances that force us to do things in new ways; tremors that impact eating and writing; gait changes and balance challenges that lead to using walking sticks, walkers, and rolling chairs; slowness that necessitates extra time for everyday tasks (like getting dressed, making dinner, crossing the street); and rigidity that stiffens our facial expression, stifles our smiles, and sometimes causes pain when we move. Parkinson's wants us to give up. Don't listen!

"Keep in mind what you can do to help yourself. Try new approaches to things. Take time to dress in clothes that are easy to put on and that make you feel good about how you look. Is there something you want to do tomorrow? Practice it today. Difficulty brushing your teeth? Electric toothbrushes are very affordable. Set goals for yourself. Can you improve your physical, emotional, mental, and social health? Can you learn something new that has nothing to do with Parkinson's?

"The more time I spend with Parkinson's, the more thankful I am for family and friends who are not deterred by my challenges and still include me in everyday activities, often with adaptations. I've made new friends in the Parkinson's community whose insights, empathy, and tenacity help me stay involved with the world. When I am invited to a gathering or activity, I do my best to join. I usually need a pre-event nap, and I might cut out early, but I give my best effort to show up.

"Stay social and stay engaged with your community. Figure out ways to let people help you. You might not think you need it now, *but your friends need everyday ways to show you they care and to stay in touch. If you stay connected now, you will all be comfortable being together when a primary care partner needs a break.*

"Parkinson's is an uninvited tagalong on all my walks—in nature, at the mall, in the grocery store—sometimes bringing on a muscle cramp so severe I crumble to the ground to wait it out (on the pavement, in the shoe store, in the frozen foods). Parkinson's comes along out to dinner, bringing dyskinesia that bothers the adjacent table so much that they ask me to stop jiggling their table. Sometimes strangers are annoyed by my Parkinson's when they have to wait for me to get out of their way, like when I try to get money from my wallet at the grocery checkout or when I don't jump aside for a runner to pass on the park's walking path. My dog is smart enough to seize the opportunity to enjoy the slow-motion moment: sniff, sniff, sniff.

"It hasn't been as bad as I thought. I know the road ahead is going to be strange. I know there will be obstacles I can't predict. We can surrender before obstacles or we can triumph little by little, day by day. There will be a cure for Parkinson's. Think about penicillin, pasteurization, x-rays, iron lungs, cardiac pacemakers, bone marrow transplants.

While I wait, I choose to do what I can to help myself and others live well, be myself, and participate in the world.

I have Parkinson's. It doesn't have me."

CHAPTER 14

Planning for Your Future

Managing Your Personal Affairs

Laurie Hanson, JD

We all know in theory that we should plan for unexpected family emergencies such as the diagnosis of a chronic illness, but day-to-day matters often cause us to push this kind of planning to the bottom of our to-do list. Planning for emergencies by necessity involves difficult family discussions we might prefer to avoid. Addressing difficult family decisions before an emergency arises is usually far easier, however, than coping with them as it is happening.

To illustrate, consider the following example:

John visited his aging mother, Bertha, and they discussed the importance of an advance directive and a power of attorney. Bertha insisted that she did not want the family to take any unusual life-prolonging measures if she could not make decisions for herself. She asked that John handle her finances if she were to become unable to do so. After this conversation, John made an appointment with his mother's attorney, and, after several more discussions among the three of them, Bertha decided to sign an advance directive and a durable power of attorney. A month later, Bertha had a severe stroke that left her unable to communicate.

If John had not started this discussion with his mother about making decisions and managing her affairs if she could not, Bertha's other children might never have learned about her end-of-life wishes. Had John and Bertha not taken the time to have an advance directive and power of attorney discussed, drafted, and signed, John would not have been able to handle even routine financial matters for his mother after her stroke. He most likely would have had to obtain a court order to get authority to manage her affairs.

This chapter explains the importance of planning for the future and provides useful information to assist you and your family. You will learn ways to ensure that your affairs are managed as you want them to be managed—even if you are no longer able to communicate or make decisions yourself.

The chapter addresses the following topics:

- Informal arrangements with friends or family
- Formal arrangements with or without court involvement
  - Managing your financial affairs using powers of attorney, trusts, and conservatorships
  - Managing your health care using advance directives; living wills; physician orders for life-sustaining treatment (POLST); do not resuscitate/do not intubate/do not hospitalize (DNR/DNI/DNH) orders; or guardianships
- Ensuring that your postdeath wishes regarding your property and the disposition of your body are followed

Your Emergency Notebook

A first step in planning for emergencies is assembling and maintaining key health, financial, and other information and documents in one place so that family members and caregivers can access the information if you are suddenly unable to communicate with them. Many organizations have developed free planning guides, but you can also create your own emergency notebook with a three-ring binder and a set of divider tabs. Organize your emergency notebook as follows, with tabs separating documents into the following sections:

1. Emergency contact information
   - Spouse, partner, or significant other
   - Children
   - Siblings
   - Parents
2. Financial and legal contact information
   - Estate attorney
   - Accountant
   - Investment advisor
3. Medical information
   - Medications (recent, past, and present)
   - Contact information for both primary care and specialist physicians
   - Immunization records
   - Significant medical, dental, and eye care details (including the physicians' names and locations of medical records)
   - Allergies
   - Significant family medical history
4. Financial information
   - Bank accounts
   - Insurance policies
   - Retirement plans
   - Stocks and bonds
   - Recurring bills (e.g., utilities, insurance, mortgage payments)
   - Real and personal property
   - Loans (receivable and payable)
   - Financial powers of attorney
   - Taxes (location of past tax returns and information for current tax year)
   - Safe deposit box

5. End-of-life information
   - Will and any accompanying statement concerning final arrangements for personal property
   - Advance directive
   - Organ donor information
   - Funeral and burial guidance
6. Location of key items
   - Important documents (e.g., passport, military records, deeds, marriage license, Social Security number, titles to vehicles)
   - Photos
   - Jewelry
7. Passwords for online accounts, mobile devices, and computers. Passwords are vital, and given that they frequently change, don't forget to update your emergency notebook, even if by hand. Passwords might be needed to access the following:
   - Email accounts, particularly those that you use to receive important medical and financial information
   - Home and office computers
   - Software programs, websites, and mobile phone apps
   - Facebook and similar social media sites (consider providing direction about how you want these handled after your death)

Many people now save all their passwords in a password manager app. Of course, it is critical that the password for the password manager mobile phone app is included in your emergency notebook.

Of course, an emergency notebook is not helpful if family members cannot find or access it. When discussing the contents of your emergency notebook with family members, be sure to explain where the notebook is located. Due to the sensitivity (e.g., medical records) and value (e.g., passwords for online bank accounts) of much of the information, however, you should give access to your emergency notebook only to a very small group of trusted family or friends.

Informal and Formal Arrangements

A second step in emergency planning is to make arrangements for anticipated and unanticipated events. Depending on the circumstances, the arrangements made will be either informal or formal.

Informal Care Arrangements

Informal arrangements are temporary and can usually be made with family, friends, and neighbors. For example, if you have surgery scheduled and know that you will be unable to perform normal household chores while you are recuperating, you may want to line up family members or friends to assist with your medication, grocery shopping, cooking, transportation to medical appointments, or housekeeping. You may also want them to help with financial matters, such as writing checks, completing tax returns, and balancing your checkbook. Such informal arrangements are very common and, in fact, make up the majority of assistance to people who are temporarily or permanently living with disabilities.

Entrusting private financial or medical information to family members or friends, however, may result in situations that have financially or medically harmful consequences. In such cases, formal arrangements are preferable. Formal arrangements may include legal safeguards regarding supervision and record-keeping or review by an outside party to minimize the risk of exploitation by an informal caregiver. Similarly, formal arrangements may also be made to protect the caregiver, who may later be questioned regarding legitimate reimbursement for services.

Although informal arrangements are often sufficient to address your need for assistance, the day may come when more formal arrangements are needed.

Formal Financial Management Services

When planning for the future, it is important to know what financial management services are available for your individual needs. These services are listed below from least formal to most formal.

Automatic Banking and Direct Deposit

Modern banking technology, such as automatic bill payment and direct deposit, can help you with your finances. At a minimum, Social Security payments and pension income should be set up so they are deposited directly into your account. Utilities and insurance payments should also be set up for automatic withdrawal from your account. This can protect you from unintentionally discontinuing your health insurance or having your electricity shut off. It is generally wise to have only one working bank account, such as a checking account, into which income is deposited and from which monthly bills are paid.

Multiple-Name Bank Accounts

Adding a name to a bank account is an easy and effective way to allow a trusted relative or friend to provide informal help. By having access to the account, that person can help sign checks, pay bills, or transfer money between your accounts. That person can also access bank records to monitor electronic deposits, ensure that all bills are paid on time, and review monthly statements to ensure that nothing is amiss.

Several types of multiple-name bank accounts are available, each with different rules. Any type of account (e.g., savings, checking, or certificate of deposit) may be held in more than one name. Such accounts are easy to set up just by visiting the bank. You should take care to select the appropriate type of account for your situation (explained next) and to ensure that you have selected a trustworthy person to help you.

The following types of multiple-name accounts are commonly available:

Joint Account: In a joint account, any person whose name is on the account is considered a co-owner. Each named person can make deposits and withdrawals without the other person's knowledge or consent. A few things about joint accounts should be kept in mind:

- The co-owner could withdraw all your money without consequence or legal recourse.
- The co-owner's creditors could tie up the funds in the account (with a lien or attachment) until proof of your ownership of the funds is provided.
- The person's name cannot be taken off the account without that person's written approval.
- In a joint account, when one owner dies, the survivor automatically owns the account without going through probate court. This can be a benefit because the funds are immediately available to pay urgent expenses, such as funeral costs. It can also have negative consequences if the joint account holder is not your intended beneficiary.

Authorized Signer Account

An authorized signer account, or a convenience account, allows another individual to make deposits, take withdrawals, and sign your checks. The other signer's creditors cannot tie up your account. As with joint accounts, however, there is a risk that the other authorized signer could withdraw all your money from your account. Unlike a joint account, the account does not belong to the other authorized signer on your death; rather, funds in this account belong to your estate or to a named beneficiary (discussed in material that follows). The authority of the other signer ends with your death, so the other authorized signer will not be able to use the funds after your death.

Payable on Death Accounts and Beneficiary Designations

All checking, savings, investment, and retirement accounts allow you to designate to whom your account will be distributed at your death. Sometimes these accounts are called payable on death (POD) accounts. Both the beneficiary designation and the POD account allow for planning after your death, but these designations do not affect ownership during your life. The named beneficiary cannot make withdrawals or sign checks, so it is a useful way to bypass probate to give money to loved ones after your death.

Naming a Representative Payee

A representative payee is an individual or organization appointed by the US Social Security Administration, US Office of Personnel Management, US Department of Veterans Affairs, or US Railroad Retirement Board who may be charged with receiving your income, using that income to pay your current expenses, saving for your future needs, and maintaining proper records. The Social Security Administration has a Representative Payee Program with rules and regulations to protect the beneficiary of the income. Learn more about the Representative Payee Program at *ssa.gov/payee*. Your representative payee must be appointed by the Social Security Administration. A power of attorney or note from you is not good enough. Having a representative appointed provides oversight that may give you assurance that your bills and finances will be properly handled. Many professional fiduciaries and organizations serve as representative payees.

Family Caregiving Contracts

Individuals are often uncomfortable with the idea of paying family members or friends for caregiving arrangements. But, changes in the Medicaid asset transfer rules over the past 15 years, as well as the reality that caregivers must sometimes give up their day jobs to provide the necessary level of care, have made personal care contracts an attractive option. These contracts help ensure the proper level of care is met and that children (or other relatives or friends) do not have to sacrifice their own financial well-being to provide care.

Personal care contracts must, as a general rule, be in writing and state the kind and extent of services that are necessary, within reasonable terms. Because personal care contracts involve payment for services, income paid to a family caregiver through such a contract is subject to payroll and income taxes, and caregivers should consult an accountant to ensure that the income is reported properly. Tax credits are not available for parent caregiving unless the parent is the child's legal dependent.

Durable Power of Attorney

A power of attorney is an extremely important planning tool. It allows you to appoint someone to manage your financial affairs if you are unable to manage them yourself. If no power of attorney exists and it is necessary to liquidate or transfer assets or enter into real estate transactions (including those of a spouse), it may be necessary to go to court to establish a conservatorship before these matters can be resolved. Establishing a conservatorship can be costly and time consuming. Thus, everyone should have a power of attorney.

Power of Attorney Defined

A power of attorney is a written document in which you (as the "principal") appoint another person (the "attorney-in-fact" or "agent") to handle your property or finances. The power of attorney can be effective for all purposes or for a limited purpose (e.g., appointing another person to sign a deed for the sale of your home when you are unavailable). Unless it is "durable" (see next section), a power of attorney becomes ineffective if the principal becomes incapacitated and all powers of attorney terminate at the passing of the principal.

Durable Power of Attorney Defined

A durable power of attorney continues to be valid even after the principal becomes incapacitated. A durable power of attorney document must specifically state that it is durable and must contain specific language, such as "this power of attorney shall continue to be effective if I become incapacitated or incompetent." Generally, if the purpose of your power of attorney is to make sure that someone can manage your finances when you cannot, the power of attorney should be durable.

Take Care When Choosing an Attorney-in-Fact

Powers of attorney are not supervised by courts, so they can be abused if the wrong person is appointed attorney-in-fact. Although an attorney-in-fact is required by law to act in the best interest of the principal, it may be difficult to get your money back if the person you have appointed handles your affairs unwisely. Therefore, you must choose someone you trust completely—a person who will always act in your best interests.

Creating a Power of Attorney

Although power of attorney forms are available without cost on the Internet, it is best to consult an experienced attorney to create a power of attorney. Too many times, individuals sign documents they have printed off the Internet only to discover later that the documents are invalid or do not serve their purposes. This can be a very costly error because it may be necessary to have a court appoint a **conservator** to do what could have been accomplished easily with a valid power of attorney.

Safeguards to Protect You

You may trust a friend or family member to be your attorney-in-fact and feel confident that no safeguards are necessary. Another option is to hire a professional fiduciary, such as a bank trust department, to ensure that your finances are handled the way you want. Either way, consider including the following safeguards in your power of attorney:

- Require that the attorney-in-fact provide an annual or monthly accounting to you, your lawyer, an independent accountant, or a trusted family member.
- Name two attorneys-in-fact in the document and specify that they must act jointly e.g., both attorneys-in-fact must agree and both must sign checks). This can slow down your agents' ability to act, but it also can serve as a protection against one of the attorneys-in-fact acting impulsively or with bad judgment.
- Require your appointed attorney-in-fact to obtain a surety bond to cover the value of your property if the attorney-in-fact mishandles your funds.
- Appoint a successor attorney-in-fact in case the attorney-in-fact dies, becomes incompetent, or simply chooses not to act on your behalf.

Canceling or Ending a Power of Attorney

A power of attorney can be canceled or revoked at any time. Each state has specific requirements for revoking a power of attorney. Your revocation should be sent to the attorney-in-fact and to any person or institution with whom the attorney-in-fact has done business on your behalf.

Remember, a power of attorney becomes invalid if the principal becomes incompetent or dies. A durable power of attorney, on the other hand, continues if the principal becomes incompetent and can be revoked only by a guardian or conservator, if one has been appointed. A durable power of attorney terminates when the principal dies.

Trusts

A trust is a legal arrangement in which a person or a financial institution owns and manages assets for your benefit. The parties to a trust are the person setting up the trust (the "grantor"), the person or organization administering the trust (the "trustee"), and the person for whom the trust is established (the "beneficiary"). Often the grantor and the beneficiary are the same person.

An agreement between the grantor and trustee, called a trust instrument, explains the trustee's authority. A trust can be created by the terms of the grantor's will (a **testamentary trust**) or during the grantor's lifetime (a **revocable trust**). A **living trust** is the type of trust used to manage assets during a time of incapacity. Some trusts are court supervised, and some are not.

Trusts are not for everyone. A living trust is generally not appropriate for modest estates because the costs and disadvantages, including the time and logistics involved in administering them, outweigh the benefits. As with any planning tool, it is important to review each option for managing estates to determine the strategies that best fit your situation. In other words, one size does not fit all.

Basic Trust Defined

You may create a trust during your lifetime by transferring ownership and control of your assets to the trustee. A trust can be revocable or irrevocable:

- As long as you are competent, you may change, revoke, or terminate a **revocable trust** at any time. A revocable trust is normally used for property management purposes. After you die, the revocable living trust becomes an irrevocable trust and can't be changed.
- A revocable living trust is often used as a planning tool because it allows a trustee to manage your property for your benefit during your life and provide for ongoing management after your incapacity or death. Most commonly, in a living trust you would be both your own trustee and beneficiary. Your Social Security number is used when establishing trust accounts or doing trust business. You would manage your property as if the property were in your name. A trust agreement would also include your directions should you become incompetent or die. If you have a medical condition that could result in your being unable to manage your affairs, a revocable living trust may be the right planning tool.
- An **irrevocable trust** cannot be changed or terminated after it has been established. It is a separate taxable entity and has its own tax identification number. Tax considerations may be a factor in deciding whether to make a trust revocable or irrevocable, particularly when a substantial amount of property is involved.

Take Care When Choosing a Trustee

A trustee has as much, if not more, responsibility as an attorney-in-fact in a power of attorney. You must take care when choosing the trustee. In most revocable living trusts, you would serve as trustee as long as you are able to do so. Should you become incapacitated, the "successor trustee" would take over and be responsible for management of all trust assets during your life and for distribution of those assets to the beneficiaries on your death. Being a trustee is a huge responsibility and should not be taken lightly. Although a family member or other individual could be named trustee if you are sure that person is trustworthy and capable of acting in this capacity, a fair amount of expertise is needed to handle the paperwork, tax returns, and property management tasks that may be involved. In most cities, professional trustees are available for hire, and many banking institutions have trust departments. Going over options with an attorney before naming a trustee is always wise.

Creating a Trust

A revocable trust is established by executing a trust agreement. In a trust agreement, you name the beneficiary (usually yourself during life), state how the property should be managed if you become disabled, and direct how the property should be distributed at your death. A revocable trust is much like a will in this way, and many states require specific formalities in signing a trust to ensure that you are not being coerced or unduly influenced by someone when executing the trust. Trusts should be drawn up by an experienced attorney.

To receive the advantages of the revocable trust, all assets must be placed in the trust or they must be jointly owned or have either a POD or beneficiary designation in them.

Important Tip

Be on guard against anyone who uses high-pressure tactics to sell a living trust package. Do not deal with anyone who demands a signature right away or requires money before you have time to do additional research. Some companies only want to sell their prepackaged plans and do not assist clients in putting assets into the trust. These trusts can cause problems that will be expensive to fix.

A Revocable Trust Cannot Be Used to Avoid Paying Nursing Home Costs

A revocable trust is considered an available resource under Medicaid laws and is not a way to avoid spending your savings on nursing home care before a state Medicaid program will begin paying those expenses. The federal and state Medicaid laws are very complicated and subject to change at any time. Do not try to use a trust in connection with asset-related nursing home care planning without getting competent legal advice.

Trusts for Protecting Assets While on Medicaid

People living with chronic conditions may ultimately require assistance with activities of daily living such as bathing, transferring, ambulation, eating, toileting, and basic hygiene and grooming. This type of assistance is known as custodial care. Individuals may receive this care at home, or they may need to move to an assisted living facility or a nursing home. No matter where these services are received, they are very expensive. Medicare does not cover the cost of custodial care. Long-term care insurance policies may cover these types of costs. It is difficult or impossible to obtain long-term care insurance after you are diagnosed with a significant medical condition, however. Also, fewer insurance companies are offering long-term care policies, and the policies still on the market are offering less coverage at a higher cost. When long-term care insurance is not available, private funds must be used to pay for the cost of care. Once private funds are depleted, many individuals turn to Medicaid to pay for these services.

Medicaid eligibility rules are complex and vary depending on a number of factors, including the state in which you reside, whether you are married or single, the types of services you need, and your age. As a general rule, however, you may keep a car and your home (as long as you are living in it) and about $2000. Be aware that this amount varies from state to state. The bottom line is that you can have only limited assets outside of your home and car.

Three types of trusts are available that, if properly established and administered, allow a person with a disability to retain more than $2000 and still be eligible for Medicaid to pay for the cost of care. These are a first-party special needs trust, a third-party special needs trust, and a pooled trust. The funds in any of these three trusts may be used to purchase goods and services that "supplement and do not supplant" government benefits. In other words, funds in the trust may be used for goods and services that benefit the individual and do not replace the government benefits the individual receives. For instance, funds may be used to pay for a companion dog, nonconventional treatments, massages, companion services, a home, rent, travel, or clothing because none of these items are covered by government benefit programs. Funds may not be used to pay for medical services covered by Medicaid. The funds held in these three types of trust do not count toward the limit on assets that applies to be eligible for Medicaid. Therefore, having a special needs trust can make a significant difference in your life. For example, sometimes a special needs trust can make the difference between living at home or in a nursing home.

It is important to understand that these three types of trusts are only available to individuals who have a disability as certified by the US Social Security Administration.

First-Party Special Needs Trust

A first-party special needs trust is a way for an individual with a disability to place his or her own money into a trust and remain eligible for Medicaid. It is called a "first-party" special needs trust because the individual's assets are used to fund the trust. Assets in a first-party special needs trust remain exempt if the trust meets the strict guidelines of the federal statute governing these trusts:

- The trust must be established by the individual with a disability or by his or her parent, grandparent, or guardian or by the court
  - For the sole benefit of the person with the disability as certified by the Social Security Administration;
  - For a person who is under the age of 65; and
  - Using the person's assets—this includes any assets a person may be awarded as a result of a personal injury lawsuit.
- The trust is irrevocable by the beneficiary and may only be changed by the trustee if the change is necessary to comply with a new law or decision governing first-party special needs trusts.
- The trust provides that at the death of the person with the disability, any remaining trust assets must be distributed first to the state as repayment for any Medicaid that has been received.

Third-Party Special Needs Trust

A third-party special needs trust is a way for a third party to give money to a person with a disability in a way that does not jeopardize the individual's eligibility for public benefits. For instance, if a parent or grandparent or best friend wants to leave money to a person with a disability, or if friends want to throw a fundraiser, a third-party special needs trust is used. Sometimes a third-party trust is set up while the grantor is alive. Alternatively, it can be set up through a will. Assets or funds belonging to the person with the disability must never be placed in the trust. There is no payback for Medicaid benefits received. Rather, the grantor states in the trust agreement who will receive any funds remaining in trust at the beneficiary's death. Laws regarding supplemental needs trusts vary from state to state, so it is important to consult with an experienced lawyer to establish a third-party special needs trust.

Pooled Special Needs Trust

A pooled trust is a type of special needs trust is administered like a first-party special needs trust. Assets in a pooled special needs trust do not count toward eligibility for public benefit programs. The only difference between the two is that a pooled trust must be established and managed by a nonprofit corporation. A separate subaccount is maintained for each beneficiary of the trust, but, for purposes of investment and management, the pooled trust aggregates the funds in all the subaccounts. Each subaccount must be established solely for the benefit of individuals who are disabled as defined by the Social Security Administration. The subaccount may be set up by the parent, grandparent, or legal guardian of the individual; the individual himself or herself; or a court. If any money remains in the subaccount at the beneficiary's death and this money is not retained by the pooled trust, the trust must use the money to reimburse the state for any Medicaid paid on behalf of the deceased beneficiary.

Healthcare Directives

An advance directive, sometimes called a health care directive, is a written document in which you appoint someone (a healthcare agent) to make healthcare decisions in the event you are unable to make them yourself.

An advance directive is essentially a combination of two documents: the living will (a document that provides specific guidance to physicians, nurses, and caregivers about medical treatment) and a durable power of attorney for health care (a document that authorizes another person to make health care decisions when you are unable to do so). Some states retain the distinction between these two types of documents, however, so it is important to know what your state's law requires.

Why Have an Advance Directive?

You have a constitutionally protected right to make decisions about your health care, including the right to refuse treatment, authorize treatment, and access information in your medical records. In a healthcare directive, you can provide directions concerning what medical treatments you do and do not want. You can also authorize a trusted loved one, relative, or caregiver (the designated healthcare agent) to make necessary healthcare decisions according to your wishes if you are unable to do so yourself.

Who Can Be a Healthcare Agent?

Your healthcare agent may be any individual 18 years of age or older who is not your healthcare provider or an employee of your healthcare provider. You should choose someone who you know well and trust to make decisions according to your wishes. It is very important to discuss your wishes in detail with a prospective healthcare agent before you name your agent. Make sure the person clearly understands your wishes and appreciates the responsibilities involved. You should also name a successor (backup) healthcare agent in case the primary healthcare agent is unable to act when decisions must be made. Both your agent and your successor agent should be individuals who will advocate in your behalf and make sure that your healthcare preferences are followed by medical providers.

What Should a Healthcare Directive Include?

Healthcare directives are governed by state law, and most state laws have several statutory requirements. Usually, state laws say that a healthcare directive must be written by a competent person and dated, signed, and witnessed or notarized.

In your healthcare directive, you may

- Appoint one or more agents or alternative agents and include instructions for how decisions should be made and whether named agents must act together or may act independently
- State a preferred nursing home in the event such care is necessary
- State which medical records the healthcare agent can access
- State that the healthcare agent is the "personal representative" under the federal Health Insurance Portability and Accountability Act (HIPAA) and has the authority to access your medical records
- State that you want your healthcare agent to become your guardian if a petition is filed
- State whether your eyes, tissues, or organs should be donated on your death
- Make a declaration regarding intrusive mental health treatment or a statement that the healthcare agent is authorized to give consent for such treatment
- State specific instructions if you are female and pregnant
- Give instructions regarding artificially administered nutrition or hydration
- State under what circumstances the healthcare directive will become effective
- State any other instructions regarding care, including how religious beliefs may affect healthcare delivery
- Provide instructions about being placed on a ventilator, receiving resuscitation, or other aggressive measures if there is minimal to no chance that you will recover
- State what will happen to your body at death (body identification/burial/cremation)

When Do the Healthcare Agent's Responsibilities Begin?

Generally, the healthcare agent may make decisions for you when your physician believes you are unable to make your own decisions. In some states, however, a healthcare agent can make decisions even if the principal has capacity, if the directive so provides.

What Are the Duties of the Healthcare Agent?

The healthcare agent is required to make informed, good-faith healthcare decisions from your point of view. The healthcare agent should follow your guidance in the healthcare directive and should seek legal help if the medical providers will not comply with his or her requests.

Can the Healthcare Directive Be Canceled or Revoked?

You may cancel or revoke the healthcare directive in whole or in part by

- Destroying the document
- Executing a written and dated statement explaining what part of the healthcare directive you want to revoke
- Orally expressing the intent to revoke it in the presence of witnesses
- Executing a new healthcare directive

Where Should the Healthcare Directive Be Kept?

The healthcare directive must be readily available in an emergency. You should keep it with your personal papers in a safe place, such as in your emergency notebook. It should not be placed in a safe deposit box because this makes the document hard to access in an emergency situation. You should give signed copies to your family members, close friends, healthcare agent, backup healthcare agent, and doctors so that they can include it in your medical records.

What Is the Uniform Anatomical Gift Act?

The Uniform Anatomical Gift Act, some version of which has been adopted in all states, allows you to donate your entire body, organs, tissues, or eyes for research or transplantation. The act also provides that if you do not make the gift, close relatives, a guardian, a conservator, or a healthcare agent may make an anatomical gift at the time of death—unless it is documented that you refused to donate organs while alive. Verification of intent to make an anatomical gift may be indicated on your driver's license.

Is a DNR/DNI/DNH the Same as a Healthcare Directive?

The acronym DNR/DNI/DNH means "do not resuscitate/do not intubate/do not hospitalize." This is a request by a patient to his or her physician to limit the scope of emergency medical care. The document making this request is signed by the patient or the patient's proxy, and it must be ordered by a physician. It will be followed by emergency medical personnel if presented to them at the time of the emergency. You should have a healthcare directive as well because the DNR/DNI/ DNH is limited only to decisions regarding end of life and resuscitation or intubation. Unlike a healthcare directive, it does not deal with the myriad healthcare issues that may arise during a medical emergency or at the end of one's life (see examples in section What Should a Healthcare Directive Include?).

What Is POLST and Is It the Same as a Healthcare Directive?

The acronym POLST stands for physician orders for life-sustaining treatment. Sometimes orders are called MOLST (medical orders for life-sustaining treatment). The POLST movement is an initiative that began in Oregon in 1991 on the theory that patient wishes for life-sustaining treatments were not being honored despite the availability of advance directives. POLST has endorsed programs in about 18 states and programs under development in most other states. Some health-care providers consider a POLST to be an important corollary to an advance directive because it is a signed medical order that is designed to be portable, specific to the patient's medical conditions, and easy for medical professionals to understand in emergency situations. Most important, it contains clear directions about the kind of intensive medical interventions a patient does or does not want initiated. Because it is a medical order, in most (but not all) states, a physician must meet with the patient to go over the form and discuss treatment options available for the specific disease or illness at issue. But, as with a DNR/DNI/DNH order, a POLST is not meant to take the place of an advance directive or the appointment of a healthcare agent.

Where Can I Obtain Healthcare Directive Forms?

An attorney who specializes in elder law or has experience with health-care directives can prepare a directive that is tailored to your needs.

In addition, suitable forms may be downloaded from reputable websites, such as the following:

- Aging with Dignity: *fivewishes.org*
- American Bar Association: *americanbar.org/groups/law_aging/ resources/health_care_decision_making/Stateforms*
- National Hospice and Palliative Care Organization: *nhpco.org/ patients-and-caregivers/*

- US Advance Care Planning Registry: *usacpr.net/individuals-families/forms-list*
- The Department of Health in individual states

Guardianship and Conservatorship

Guardianships and conservatorships are relationships between two people created by the court to protect individuals who cannot handle their own financial or personal affairs. Definitions vary from state to state. Generally, a **guardian** is appointed for the purpose of managing the personal affairs of a person who has become incapacitated (called a ward), including making personal decisions and meeting needs for medical care, nutrition, clothing, shelter, or safety. A **conservator** is appointed for a person (called a protected person) for the purpose of managing finances, assets, and income when it has been shown that the person has impaired ability or judgment. If a person needs both a guardian and a conservator, one person may be appointed by the court to fill both of those roles.

When Is a Guardianship or Conservatorship Required?

A guardianship or conservatorship is necessary when a person becomes unable to handle finances or live safely without help and no previous arrangements have been made. The decision to obtain a guardianship or conservatorship should not be made lightly because it takes away the person's most basic right: to make decisions about his or her own health and welfare. The court will appoint a guardian or conservator who will handle most or all of the person's affairs, including perhaps where he or she will live.

The court will appoint a guardian or conservator only if a less restrictive alternative is not available for managing the personal and financial affairs of the person. Courts are much less likely to approve a guardianship or conservatorship if a healthcare directive and a power of attorney have been put into place.

Establishment of a Guardianship or Conservatorship

Although specific practices may vary state by state, generally a guardianship or conservatorship is established by filing a petition with the probate court in the county where the person resides. Anyone over the age of 18 can ask the court to appoint a guardian or conservator for a person who needs help. The potential ward or protected person must be given advance notice of the hearing and, in most states, has the right to be represented by an attorney at any court proceeding, even if he or she cannot pay for the attorney. The person requesting a guardianship or conservatorship must prove through clear and convincing evidence that such an order is necessary. This could be difficult if the proposed ward or protected person does not want a guardianship or conservatorship established.

Your Will

A will is a set of written instructions about how to dispose of your assets upon death. Assets are described as either probate assets or nonprobate assets. Probate assets are those assets whose ownership a court must rule on following the owner's death. Nonprobate assets are assets that will automatically transfer to another person at death, such as those with joint tenancy or beneficiary designations or assets that have been placed in a trust. Probate court is the court charged with determining ownership either by administering a legal will or by state law when no legal will exists.

Not Everyone Needs a Will—But It Is a Good Idea

If all of a person's property is held in such a way that it will pass through beneficiary designations or joint ownership, then a will is not technically necessary. A will is necessary, however, if a person wants personal property, such as jewelry, paintings, and family heirlooms, distributed in a certain way. There are many reasons to have a will even if significant assets are nonprobate assets. These include tax reasons and family considerations. Finally, even if there seems to be no reason for a will, having one is the best way to ensure that an individual's wishes will be followed.

Find Out More

Support groups and advocacy groups aren't the only places to learn about Parkinson's disease. There are many free online sources and free pamphlets you can access. When searching for information on the Internet, it's important to look for websites, magazines, workbooks, and pamphlets published by trusted organizations. Here are some more resources:

Parkinson's Organizations:

American Parkinson Disease Association
800-223-2732
apdaparkinson.org

Davis Phinney Foundation for Parkinson's
866-358-0285
davisphinneyfoundation.org

Michael J. Fox Foundation for Parkinson's Research
800-708-7644
michaeljfox.org

Parkinson's Foundation
800-473-4636
parkinson.org

The Parkinson Alliance
800-579-8440
parkinsonalliance.org

Additional Resources:
American Music Therapy Association
301-589-3300
musictherapy.org

American Occupational Therapy Association
301-652-6611
aota.org

American Parkinson Disease Association Resource Booklets
800-223-2732
apdaparkinson.org/resources-support/download-publications/

Titles include
- *Parkinson's Disease Handbook—New Edition*
- *Be Active & Beyond—A Guide to Exercise and Wellness for People with Parkinson's Disease—New Edition*
- *Helping Those Who Serve: Parkinson's Disease Information for the Veterans Community*
- *Make Your Voice Heard! Healthy Communication and Parkinson's Disease*
- *My Mommy Has Parkinson's Disease But It's Okay!—New Edition*

American Physical Therapy Association
800-999-2782
apta.org

American Speech-Language-Hearing Association
800-638-8255
asha.org

Brain & Life
646-674-6545
brainandlife.org

A free website and bimonthly print magazine published by the American Academy of Neurology; it includes many articles on Parkinson's disease and related therapies.

Eldercare Locator, Administration on Aging, an agency of the US Administration for Community Living
800-677-1116
eldercare.acl.gov/Public/Index

Family Caregiver Alliance
800-445-8106
www.caregiver.org

Job Accommodation Network, Office of Disability and Employment Policy, US Department of Labor
800-526-7234
askjan.org

LSVT Global, Lee Silverman Voice Treatment (LSVT) LOUD and BIG
888-438-5788
lsvtglobal.com

Melvin Weinstein Parkinson's Foundation
757-313-9729
mwpf.org

Caregiver Action Network
855-227-3640
caregiveraction.org

National Sleep Foundation: Parkinson's Disease and Sleep
703-243-1697
sleepfoundation.org/articles/parkinsons-disease-and-sleep

Parkinson's Foundation Resource Books
800-473-4636
parkinson.org/pd-library

A variety of books and fact sheets, including

- *Aware in Care* (a toolkit for hospitalization)
- *Caring and Coping*
- *Fitness Counts*
- *Guide to Deep Brain Stimulation*
- *Managing Parkinson's Mid-Stride: A Treatment Guide to Parkinson's*
- *Mood: A Mind Guide to Parkinson's Disease*
- *Parkinson's Medications: Today and Tomorrow*
- *Speech and Swallowing*
- *Psychosis: A Mind Guide to Parkinson's Disease*
- *What You and Your Family Should Know*

Parkinson Wellness Recovery
520-591-5346
pwr4life.org

Rock Steady Boxing
rocksteadyboxing.org

GLOSSARY

Acetylcholine One of the neurotransmitters.

Adrenaline A hormone produced by the adrenal glands (small glands sitting on top of the kidneys). This chemical is used by some nerve cells of the autonomic nervous system to communicate with organs such as the heart, the gut, the skin, and the pupil of the eye.

Agoraphobia A condition in which a person becomes very anxious or panicky in crowded situations or on being outside his or her home.

Akathisia An inability to sit still, caused by an "ants-in-the-pants" feeling. This is different from restless legs as it is not under voluntary control.

Akinesia An inability to move or initiate voluntary movement.

Antioxidants Chemicals or nutrients that scavenge free radicals, the toxic byproducts of natural chemical processes that take place inside normal or diseased cells.

Antipsychotic drugs Medications used to control psychotic symptoms (e.g., hallucinations, delusions, and paranoia).

Apathy Loss of interest, motivation, or emotional response.

Apraxia Inability of the brain to plan, initiate, and execute certain tasks or even simple voluntary movements.

Atypical parkinsonism or atypical parkinsonian syndrome A condition that resembles Parkinson's but is caused by a different disease. The term is used when evidence is insufficient to make a more precise diagnosis, such as multiple-system atrophy or progressive supranuclear palsy.

Autonomic nervous system The part of the nervous system that controls automatic or involuntary functions of the body. In simple terms, these are functions that a person doesn't have to think about, such as heartbeat, sweating, and the movements of our stomach and intestines.

Basal ganglia Clumps of nerve cells deep inside the brain whose job is to work out the details of most voluntary actions. For example, when a movement is initiated, it is the job of the basal ganglia to ensure that the movement is accurate, smooth, and performed with adequate speed.

Benign tremulous parkinsonism A form of Parkinson's disease in which patients have a lot of tremor but relatively little rigidity or bradykinesia.

Blood-brain barrier A complex system of cells in the brain that control the entry and exit of chemicals and nutrients into and out of the brain.

Bradykinesia Slowness of movement.

Bradyphrenia Slowness of thinking processes.

Camptocormia A pronounced forward lean of the trunk.

Carbidopa A medication that blocks the breakdown of levodopa outside the brain, thereby maximizing the amount of levodopa that ends up in the brain and cutting back some of its side effects, such as nausea.

Carbidopa/levodopa A pill that contains both of these medications.

CBD See *Corticobasal degeneration*.

Chorea Involuntary and uncontrollable dancelike movements.

Cognition The combined functions of the brain that have to do with the thinking processes.

Cognitive dysfunction A malfunction of the thinking processes of the brain.

COMT inhibitors A group of anti-Parkinson's drugs that work by blocking the breakdown of levodopa, thereby prolonging its effectiveness.

Conservator An individual appointed to be responsible for managing finances, assets, and income of an individual who is incapacitated (a protected person).

Corticobasal degeneration A neurodegenerative disease that shares some features with Parkinson's disease and may sometimes look like Parkinson's disease.

DaT scan See *Dopamine transporter scan.*

DBS See *Deep brain stimulation.*

Deep brain stimulation A brain surgery that introduces a wire into the brain; through the wire the activity of certain areas of the brain can be regulated to restore normal function.

Delusion An abnormal thought or idea that has no base in reality. Examples of delusions are when people think that others are after them, that they are being watched, or that their spouses are unfaithful.

Dementia Cognitive dysfunction that is sufficient to cause significant impairment in one's day-to-day activities and is not due to a reversible cause. The most well-known dementia is Alzheimer's disease, but dementia can be caused by many diseases, including Parkinson's disease.

Dementia with Lewy bodies A neurodegenerative disease that combines features of Parkinson's disease with early dementia.

Diplopia Double vision.

Disease modifying A term used to describe medications that may alter the course of disease progression (ideally by slowing it down).

DLB See *Dementia with Lewy bodies.*

DNA The material of which genes are composed.

Dopamine One of the neurotransmitters.

Dopamine agonist A drug that exerts its action by stimulating dopamine receptors.

Dopamine receptors Proteins through which dopamine exerts its actions.

Dopamine transporter scan (DaT scan) A brain scan that uses a radioactive tracer that identifies dopamine neurons in the brain; it can be used as one of many tests to help diagnose Parkinson's disease.

Dopaminergic Using a dopamine-related mechanism.

Dopaminergic neurons Nerve cells that produce and use dopamine to communicate.

Duodenum The first part of the small intestine, immediately downstream from the stomach.

Dys- A prefix used to mean difficult or abnormal.

Dysarthria Slurred speech.

Dysautonomia Dysfunction of the autonomic nervous system.

Dysexecutive syndrome A type of cognitive dysfunction that affects executive functions of the brain, such as planning and organizing one's actions, taking initiative, solving problems, managing different tasks simultaneously, and performing complex tasks that require multiple choreographed steps.

Dyskinesia Abnormal, involuntary movements as a side effect of medications.

Dysphagia Difficulty with swallowing.

Dysphonia Difficulty with producing a strong or clear voice.

Dystonia Abnormal, involuntary movement that results from the simultaneous contraction of muscles that have opposing actions. Dystonic movements are slow, cramped, and usually follow a repeating pattern. Alternatively, dystonia is a disease characterized predominantly by dystonic movements.

Emotional lability Inability to control emotional outbursts, such as crying or laughing with very little provocation.

Executive function The function of the brain that has to do with planning our actions, making decisions, directing our attention, stopping us from doing things we consider inappropriate, detecting and correcting mistakes, and making choices.

Exercise physiologist A professional who specializes in the use of therapeutic exercise.

Feeding tube A thin, flexible tube inserted into the stomach or the duodenum, usually through the nose and the esophagus, for the purpose of administering nutrition and medications to people who have lost their ability to swallow temporarily.

Free radicals Byproducts of normal chemical processes that occur inside cells. Free radicals can cause oxidation, permanently damaging normal components inside cells, a process that has been considered central to the aging process and cell death. Normal cells have mechanisms to prevent this damage, and some nutritional supplements and vitamins can help. These "good chemicals" are called antioxidants.

Freezing of gait A symptom in Parkinson's disease and other diseases in which one's feet feel glued to the ground.

Frequency In the context of Parkinson's disease, this usually means having to urinate frequently.

Gastrostomy A procedure in which a tube is inserted into the stomach or the duodenum through the skin of the abdomen to provide a way to administer nutrients and medications to people who have lost their ability to swallow.

Gene A portion of a cell's DNA that contains the blueprint for the cell to build a specific protein.

Genome The full list of all the genes in a species (e.g., humans, dogs, rats, or monkeys).

Globus pallidus A structure in the basal ganglia, often used as a target for deep brain stimulation surgery in Parkinson's.

Guardian A person appointed for the purpose of managing the personal affairs of an individual who is incapacitated (a ward). A guardian is responsible for making personal decisions for the ward and for meeting the ward's needs for medical care, nutrition, clothing, shelter, or safety.

Hallucination A perception of something that does not exist (e.g., seeing dead people or hearing music that's not there).

Healthcare directive A written document, often also referred to as an advance directive, in which an individual appoints someone (a healthcare agent) to make healthcare decisions in the event that the individual cannot make them independently and to give instructions regarding health care.

Hereditary Transmitted through the genes.

Hoehn and Yahr scale A staging system for Parkinson's disease.

Hyper- A prefix used to mean increased, excessive, or enhanced.

Hypersomnia Excessive sleepiness.

Hypo- A prefix used to mean decreased, deficient, or suppressed.

Hypokinesia (adjective hypokinetic) Decreased mobility or movement.

Illusion Misinterpretation of sensory stimuli. For example, a person might look at a bush and misinterpret it as a person crouching.

Insomnia Sleeplessness.

Irrevocable trust A trust that may not be changed or terminated after it has been established. It is a separate taxable entity, requiring its own tax identification number.

Jejunum The second part of the small intestines, immediately downstream from the duodenum.

L-Dopa See *Levodopa*.

Lee Silverman Voice Treatment A specialized speech therapy program to improve voice in Parkinson's patients.

Levodopa A drug that is the raw material for making dopamine.

Lewy body A collection of damaged proteins inside nerve cells affected by Parkinson's disease.

Lewy body disease A neurodegenerative disease with many similarities to Parkinson's that has additional symptoms, such as early symptoms of dementia and hallucinations.

Living trust A trust created during the grantor's lifetime.

LSVT See *Lee Silverman Voice Treatment.*

Magnetic resonance imaging A scan of the brain using a high-power magnetic field.

MAO-B inhibitors A class of anti-Parkinson's medications that block one of the enzymes that breaks down dopamine.

Micrographia A symptom of Parkinson's disease in which handwriting becomes small and difficult to read.

Mild cognitive impairment (MCI) Cognitive dysfunction that is greater than expected for a person's age but not sufficiently severe to qualify as dementia (see *Dementia*).

Mitochondria Components of cells that specialize in extracting energy from oxygen.

Motor symptoms Symptoms having to do with movement and mobility.

Movement disorders specialist A neurologist who specializes in Parkinson's disease and other diseases that affect mobility and movement, such as dystonia and chorea.

MPTP A chemical that kills dopamine neurons and can cause a Parkinson's-like illness in people and monkeys.

MRI See *Magnetic resonance imaging.*

Multidisciplinary model of care A care model in which specialists from multiple therapeutic disciplines work together to help people with Parkinson's and their families better manage living with the disease.

Multiple system atrophy A neurodegenerative disease that combines features of Parkinson's with early and prominent dysautonomia or ataxia (a motor dysfunction similar to being drunk).

Myoclonus Sudden, jerky, fast, and unpredictable involuntary movements.

Neurodegenerative Related to premature death of neurons that does not result from a specific cause, such as injury, chemicals, tumors, or strokes.

Neurogenic bladder Urinary bladder dysfunction that results from a disease of the nervous system.

Neurologist A medical specialist who specializes in diseases of the nervous system.

Neuron A nerve cell.

Neuroplasticity A process through which new connections develop between neurons.

Neuroprotective Protecting nerve cells from disease-related damage or a drug that has this effect.

Neuropsychologist A psychologist who specializes in assessing cognition.

Neurosurgeon A surgeon who specializes in surgery of the brain and other nervous system structures.

Neurotoxin A poison that affects nerve cells.

Neurotransmitter 1. A naturally occurring substance produced by nerve cells used to communicate with other nerve cells or organs. Dopamine, acetylcholine, norepinephrine, serotonin, and glutamate are some of the most important neurotransmitters in the brain. 2. The "battery pack" that generates the electrical stimulation in deep brain stimulation.

Nocturia The condition of having to urinate frequently at night.

Nonmotor symptoms Symptoms that do not have to do with movement and mobility.

Norepinephrine One of the neurotransmitters.

Normal-pressure hydrocephalus A condition in which the abnormal accumulation of excess spinal fluid in the cavities of the brain (the ventricles) produces symptoms similar to those of Parkinson's disease.

Nutritionist   A healthcare professional who specializes in proper nutrition.

Occupational therapist A healthcare professional who helps people improve their abilities to perform their daily activities, from getting in and out of bed to activities such as bathing, showering, writing, cooking, using utensils, and improving hand dexterity.

On/off phenomenon The occurrence of mostly unpredictable spells during which anti-Parkinson's drugs lose their effectiveness.

Orthostatic hypotension (or postural hypotension) A significant drop in one's blood pressure on standing up that may lead to lightheadedness or even fainting.

Pallidotomy A type of deep brain stimulation surgery in which the stimulating electrode is placed in the globus pallidus.

Pallidum See *Globus pallidus.*

Parkin A protein in neurons; mutations in the gene that is responsible for producing this protein causes a genetic form of Parkinson's.

Parkinson's disease A neurodegenerative disease characterized by the loss of dopamine neurons in the substantia nigra.

Parkinson's disease dementia (PDD) Dementia that may occur in the advanced stages of Parkinson's disease.

Parkinson's disease psychosis Hallucinations and delusions that may happen as a result of progression of Parkinson's disease.

Parkinsonism A constellation of symptoms similar to those of Parkinson's disease. Many diseases and some drugs can cause parkinsonism without causing Parkinson's disease.

Pathologist A doctor specializing in pathology (see next definition).

Pathology Abnormal changes that happen in tissues, organs, and cells as a result of illness or injury. Also, the medical specialty that deals with investigating such changes.

PDD See *Parkinson's disease dementia.*

Percutaneous endoscopic gastrostomy A procedure to provide a way to administer nutrients and medications to people who have lost the ability to swallow. A tube is inserted into the stomach or the duodenum through the skin of the abdomen with the aid of a flexible "telescope" inserted in the stomach through the mouth and the esophagus.

Peripheral neuropathy (or polyneuropathy) A condition in which the nerves that convey messages from the spinal cord to the muscles and other organs and also bring information back to the spinal cord and brain (including sensations such as touch, pain, and temperature) are damaged.

Personalized medicine   According to the US Food and Drug Administration, " 'Personalized medicine' may be thought of as tailoring medical treatment to the individual characteristics, needs, and preferences of each patient. 'Personalized medicine' is not limited to pharmaceutical therapy. Advances in computational power and medical imaging are paving the way for personalized medical treatments that consider a patient's genetic, anatomical, and physiological characteristics."

Physical therapist A healthcare professional who helps patients with mobility, balance, or musculoskeletal problems through specific therapies and exercises and through other nonmedication treatments, such as ultrasound, heat application, and special equipment.

Pisa syndrome A sideways leaning of the trunk.

Placebo A "dummy" pill that contains no active drug but looks and tastes the same as one that does.

Positron emission tomography (PET) An advanced brain scan that maps the function and chemistry of the different parts of the brain.

Postural instability A decline in one's ability to remain standing without losing his or her balance.

Power of attorney A written document in which an individual (the principal) appoints another person (the attorney-in-fact) to handle property or finances.

Progressive supranuclear palsy A neurodegenerative disease that can look very much like Parkinson's, especially in its early stages.

Proteasome A component of cells that recycles old or damaged proteins.

PSP See *Progressive supranuclear palsy.*

Psychiatrist A medical specialist who diagnoses and treats diseases that present with emotional and behavioral symptoms, such as depression, anxiety, or schizophrenia.

Psychologist A healthcare professional who diagnoses and treats psychiatric disorders through nonmedication therapies.

Psychosis A disorder in which patients have altered perceptions of reality. Examples include paranoia and schizophrenia.

RBD See *REM sleep behavior disorder.*

Receptors Protein molecules on the surface of nerve cells that act as switches for the electrical activity of the cell.

REM sleep behavior disorder A sleep disorder in which affected persons act out their dreams.

Restless legs syndrome A condition in which a person has an uncomfortable sensation in his or her legs while sitting or reclining. The condition is often relieved by getting up and walking.

Revocable trust A type of trust normally used for property management purposes. Such a trust may be changed, revoked, or terminated at any time during the lifetime of an individual as long as he or she is competent. After death, a revocable trust becomes irrevocable.

Rigidity Muscle stiffness.

Sensory symptoms Abnormal sensations of numbness, tingling, pain, or changes in vision, hearing, taste, or smell.

Serotonin One of the neurotransmitters.

Social worker A professional who can assist patients with understanding insurance and disability issues, getting help in the community, and finding the right living situation (e.g., assisted living or a nursing home).

Speech pathologist (also speech language pathologist) A healthcare professional who provides therapies for speech, voice, and swallowing problems.

Stereotaxic (or stereotactic) surgery A type of brain surgery where a sophisticated technique is used to place probes or wires in deep parts of the brain with great precision and without extensive cutting through the brain.

Striatum One of the basal ganglia structures.

Substantia nigra The basal ganglia structure that contains the dopamine neurons.

Subthalamic nucleus A structure in the basal ganglia, often used as a target for deep brain stimulation surgery in Parkinson's.

α-Synuclein A protein in found in neurons; mutations in the gene that is responsible for producing this protein cause a genetic form of Parkinson's. α-Synuclein is one of the proteins that accumulate in Lewy bodies.

Testamentary trust A trust created by the terms of the grantor's will.

Thalamotomy A surgical procedure used to control tremor. It consists of making a controlled small lesion, like a ministroke, in a part of the brain called the thalamus to "reset" the circuits in the brain that are responsible for the generation of the tremors.

Thalamus A cluster of cells in the deep parts of the brain with many relay functions, including transmission of motor and sensory signals. It can be seen as the central switchboard of the brain.

Tremor Involuntary rhythmic shaking of a limb.

Ubiquitin A protein found in neurons; ubiquitin is one of the proteins that accumulate in Lewy bodies.

Unified Parkinson's Disease Rating Scale A scale used to rate the severity of Parkinson's symptoms.

UPDRS See *Unified Parkinson's Disease Rating Scale.*

Urgency A sensation that one has to urinate immediately.

Video swallowing assessment A modified x-ray that assesses the swallowing function.

Wearing off The loss of anti-Parkinson's effect toward the end of the interval between medication doses.

Will A set of written instructions outlining how an individual wishes to have her or his assets distributed on death.

ABOUT THE AUTHORS AND CONTRIBUTORS

Sotirios A. Parashos, MD, PhD, Lead Physician for Clinical Research, Struthers Parkinson's Center, HealthPartners Park Nicollet, Golden Valley, Minnesota; Associate Consultant Neurologist, Park Nicollet Clinic, St. Louis Park, Minnesota, and Struthers Parkinson's Center, HealthPartners, St. Paul, Minnesota; Core Faculty, Allied Team Training Program Parkinson's Foundation; Adjunct Professor of Neurology, University of Minnesota, Minneapolis, Minnesota.

Rose L. Wichmann, PT, Director of Parkinson's Programs, Struthers Parkinson's Center, HealthPartners Park Nicollet, Golden Valley, Minnesota.

Sierra Farris, PA-C, MPAS, Neurological Physician Assistant, Deep Brain Stimulation Specialist, Author.

Laurie Hanson, JD, Shareholder with Long, Reher, & Hanson, PA, an elder law firm in Minneapolis, Minnesota, established to represent individuals and family members who are aging or living with disabilities. Ms. Hanson concentrates her practice exclusively in disability planning. Ms. Hanson is a member of the National Academy of Elder Law Attorneys and the Special Needs Alliance, a national professional association of attorneys committed to helping individuals with disabilities, their families, and the professionals who represent them.

Susan Imke, FNP, GNP-C, Nurse Practitioner, Kane Hall Barry Neurology, Bedford, Texas; Advisory Board Member, Parkinson Alliance; Allied Team Training Program, National Parkinson Foundation; Educational Consultant, American Parkinson Disease Association.

Martha A. Nance, MD, Medical Director, Struthers Parkinson's Center, Park Nicollet Methodist Hospital, Golden Valley, Minnesota; Consultant Neurologist, Park Nicolet Clinic, St. Louis Park, Minnesota; Adjunct Professor of Neurology, University of Minnesota, Minneapolis, Minnesota.

Ergun Y. Uc, MD, Professor of Neurology; Director, Division of Movement Disorders, Department of Neurology, University of Iowa, Iowa City, Iowa; Director, Parkinson's Foundation Center of Excellence at the University of Iowa; Associate Editor, *Parkinsonism & Related Disorders*.

ABOUT THE AMERICAN ACADEMY
OF NEUROLOGY

Founded in 1948, the American Academy of Neurology now represents more than 36,000 members who are neurologists and neuroscience professionals and is dedicated to promoting the highest quality patient-centered neurologic care. A neurologist is a doctor with specialized training in diagnosing, treating, and managing disorders of the brain and nervous system such as Alzheimer's disease, stroke, migraine, multiple sclerosis, concussion, Parkinson's disease, and epilepsy.

For more information about the American Academy of Neurology, visit *Aan.com*.

To sign up for a print or digital free subscription to *Brain & Life*®, the American Academy of Neurology's magazine for patients and caregivers, visit *Brainandlife.org*.

INDEX

Figures and boxes are indicated by *f* and *b* following the page number
For the benefit of digital users, indexed terms that span two pages
(e.g., 52–53) may, on occasion, appear on only one of those pages.